Art Therapy and Emotion Regulation Problems

Suzanne Haeyen

Art Therapy and Emotion Regulation Problems

Theory and Workbook

palgrave
macmillan

Suzanne Haeyen
HAN University of Applied Sciences
Nijmegen, The Netherlands

and

GGNet, Mental Health Care Institute and
Scelta, Expert Centre Personality Disorders
Nijmegen/Apeldoorn, The Netherlands

Translated by C. L. Stennes, Amsterdam, The Netherlands

ISBN 978-3-030-07248-3 ISBN 978-3-319-96773-8 (eBook)
https://doi.org/10.1007/978-3-319-96773-8

Cover illustration: Caroline, client, 27
Cover design: Fatima Jamadar

This Palgrave Macmillan imprint is published by the registered company Springer Nature Switzerland AG
The registered company address is: Gewerbestrasse 11, 6330 Cham, Switzerland

Foreword I

Dialectical Behavior Therapy (DBT) was developed by Prof. Marsha Linehan for treating chronically suicidal patients diagnosed with borderline personality disorder (BPD). Since its development, DBT has been extensively researched. It has proven to be an effective treatment for a wide array of mental disorders. The treatment components and treatment strategies are rooted in Linehan's biosocial theory (1993). Linehan states that the transaction between emotional vulnerability and an invalidating social environment results in pervasive emotion dysregulation. The main focus of DBT is helping patients to get out of this vicious circle and take realisable steps in the direction of a life worth living.

DBT combines weekly individual cognitive–behavioural psychotherapy sessions with the primary therapist, weekly skills-training groups lasting 2–2.5 hours per week, as needed consultation for the patients, and weekly consultation meetings for the trainers and therapists (Linehan, 2002). Individual therapy focuses primarily on motivational issues, including the motivation to stay alive and to stay in treatment. The first phase of the treatment is learning new skills in order to stop the vicious circle of emotion dysregulated behaviours, negative outcomes and invalidation from the environment.

The specific working mechanism of DBT is motivating patients to practice the DBT skills. Making more use of the skills precedes a decrease in suicidal, nonsuicidal self-injury (NSSI) and depression. Making less use of the skills increases the chance of drop-out, even if common treatment processes are accounted for. Applying the skills gives the individual the possibility to observe the situation, to get a grip on what is happening, and to experience emotions without having to act upon them.

In other words, DBT has fostered hope. Mental health care therapists believe that treatment, even of the most severe personality problems like suicidality or self-destructive behaviour, is possible. The diagnosis of personality disorder or BPD has become less of a lifetime sentence. However, implementation of the guidelines for treatment of personality disorders has shown to be difficult.

One of the difficulties, especially in residential treatment settings, is merging an evidence-based treatment like DBT with practice-based non-verbal treatments like art therapy. Many therapists and patients have experienced the benefits of a combination of verbal-based treatment approaches and non-verbal therapy. However, research results are scarce. In this era of cost-effectiveness, lack of data poses a threat to non-verbal therapies. Insurance companies and policy-makers may falsely interpret a lack of data as evidence for the opinion that non-verbal therapies are not effective or not clinically meaningful.

This is where this book comes in. Suzanne Haeyen shows the added value of art therapy in daily practice and in numbers. Using a lot of DBT-based skills, the author stipulates how she helps individuals diagnosed with PD's in general and BPD in specific to gain insight into their emotions and actions. Art helps individuals to experience emotions and to explore their meaning. Her research that has been published in several articles shows that art therapy not only decreases symptoms of psychopathology of personality disorders, but also leads to a more optimal personal performance, self-acceptance and in strengthening the ability to experience a higher level of well-being.

Finally, the book also shows how art therapy can enhance cognitive skills as described in the part about schema-focused therapy.

I believe that this book needs to be part of the library of every therapist that treats individuals with BPD.

Suzanne explains how art therapy can help patients to communicate emotions when words cannot (yet) be found. One of the moving examples in which she shows what happens to patients is described in chapter six. 'You can try to find the words, but I couldn't connect, my vocabulary was just not appropriate [...] I am very rational and analytical, but it doesn't bring me any closer to my feelings. In art therapy, you don't use words, but you feel things, literally. It happened earlier, when we were working on the circles with the rational mind, the emotional mind and the wise mind. I was working with chalk on the emotional circle, I felt huge emotions rise in me, and I had to cry. There and then, I just wanted to leave off drawing, I wanted some attention and wanted to talk about it, but I was left on my own... The therapist told me that I could just let the feelings be there, and so I thought, "okay, let them be there", and that was a breakthrough'.

And this, as we know, opens the door to inner wisdom, compassion, and ultimately a life worth living.

Apeldoorn, The Netherlands/Belgium

Wies van den Bosch
President DBT

References

Linehan, M. M. (1993). *Cognitive-behavioral treatment of borderline personality disorder*. New York, NY: Guilford Press.

Linehan, M. M. (2002). *Dialectische gedragstherapie bij borderline persoonlijkheidsstoornis: theorie en behandeling*. Lisse: Swets & Zeitlinger.

Foreword II

Thinking about what is painful, shameful or threatening is often not easy. It is even harder to describe it to someone else. And yet each of us has the ability to look our darker sides in the eye and, together with another person, to give meaning to them in a way that creates a new outlook, greater scope. Even with the courage to take the plunge, you have no idea where you will wind up—off balance at times and sometimes even in free fall. This is offset by your own innate resilience; you only need to find it, even if you are falling. While you descend into your inner world, something else is ascending. Not just the awareness of your own strength, but also new meaning. You see what is essential in your own life, what is valuable. But it still takes perseverance to bring that insight to life. It is an exercise that may even last a lifetime.

If you accept the challenge, you take the plunge.

Many of our clients are like that. They take the plunge, but into an internalised image. It is an activity that does not require much talking. Art therapy also works primarily with images. The words will come later. To people who are not on very good terms with words, or people who cannot reach their feelings with words, it is a boon. How this works and what significance it has for clients who experience the most difficult of all mental health problems are shown by Suzanne Haeyen in this beautiful book in a highly engaging manner.

Suzanne has taken a plunge herself. If a person decides to take a deep breath and write a book like this one, she follows the entire cycle until the book has been completed and movement is no longer needed. In itself, and even before reading the book, this asks for plenteous and fitting admiration.

Warnsveld, The Netherlands

Kees Lemke
Medical Director
GGNet, Mental Health Care Institute

Acknowledgements

I want to thank everyone who contributed in any way to this book. First of all, my thanks go to Ton for his generous and loving support and his critical reading. I am grateful to my sons Ward, Luc en Boas for their pride and enthusiasm and for keeping me supplied with food and drink when they thought I had been working much too long. Thanks go to my colleagues of the teams for personality disorders of the expert centre 'Scelta' at GGNet, mental health care institute, for their contribution to the description of the multidisciplinary relationships in the various aspects of treatment. I thank Kees Lemke and Wies van den Bosch for their kind forewords. And last but certainly not least, I want to thank all the clients I have worked with, who always continue to inspire me, and particularly Katie, who was willing to tell her own story in this book.

Without all of you, this book would not be what it is today!

Suzanne Haeyen

Contents

Part II Workbook

List of Figures

Introduction

This book is about art therapy for people with emotion regulation problems. Or in more specific diagnostic terms: people diagnosed with personality disorders. It is meant to shed some light on this theme at different levels and on the basis of different frameworks. It does not intend to paint a complete picture; the field of personality disorders is a broad one.

I prefer to use the term emotion regulation problems, and these problems are often related to complex trauma. Although the diagnosis of personality disorders is regularly used, it is surrounded by controversy: many therapists and service users who feel that the diagnosis of personality disorder does not reflect their lived experience and believe that it is stigmatising. The texts and assignments in this book can be appropriate for people with many serious and long-term problems.

To delineate the target group described in this book, emphasis is on personality problems in clusters B and C and not specifically on one disorder within that area. In the field of diagnostics, for some time there have been calls to leave behind the classification of specific personality disorders because there is often an overlap between these areas, and it is closer to reality to speak of clusters or to choose a multidimensional approach.

In practice, I have encountered clients with personality issues in various parts of mental health care: in acute psychiatry, in long-term care, in specialised part-time programmes and in outpatient treatments where art therapy is offered as a plus to a verbal therapy. Over time, these experiences led me to write a number of articles on the subject which have been reworked and included in this book, with some additions and product descriptions. I chose the present structure for this book because a central thread had started to show itself, linking together the various parts.

This book was previously published in the Netherlands [Dutch title: *Niet uitleven maar beleven. Beeldende therapie bij persoonlijkheidsproblematiek*]. Since it has been published, it is very popular among art therapists in the field and art therapy students. The book is on the reading list of every educational programme for Art Therapy in the Netherlands.

Part I: The Chapters

The first chapter describes the phenomenon of personal space and how this is a basic theme in art therapy for clients with personality disorders. It is about the relationship between personality development in early childhood, how children's drawings develop and giving shape to works in art therapy by adult clients with personality disorders. Art therapy influences the client's autonomy and ego strength.

In the second chapter, art therapy with lower-level borderline clients is described and linked to the relationship management theory. The qualities of art therapy and the various aspects of the expressive medium and the art work thus created are applied to the client group.

The third chapter describes art therapy based on Linehan's dialectical behaviour therapy (DBT). Dialectics show themselves in art therapy in various ways; they are visible in the product, and they are linked to the creative process and can be found in a variety of expressive assignments that are based on polarities. Art therapy based on DBT is meant to teach people to express and regulate their emotions, to achieve a stable self-image, to work on interpersonal skills and crisis skills. Because the experience of art therapy is central, clients are better able to integrate the theory of DBT.

The fourth chapter is about Young's schema-focused therapy, which offers a framework for working in art therapy with experiential techniques such as imagery, in which concrete, personal experiences and underlying schemas can be studied. After the imagery, inner images can be shaped into external forms. This makes it possible to anchor, confirm and reflect on these inner images. This chapter is a summary of the main findings of clients who carried out an imagery exercise and then portrayed their findings in an art work. Their findings show that the objectives were attained and that the creative aspect added essential features.

The fifth chapter is about letting go and holding on in art therapy: an important theme that comes up in all manner of forms and at all levels. At an intrapsychic level, it revolves around the central questions in the therapy: What is the problem? What do I want to change? What will I have to forgo? And is that what I really want? These questions are related to the theme of transfer: What do I want to take with me and what will I let go of or leave behind? It is important to consciously encourage transfer and to devote attention to the process of holding on to the experiences gained in art therapy. Several possible interventions to achieve this are discussed.

This chapter is followed by the story of Katie, a former client who looks back at the process she went through in art therapy.

In this day and age, this book cannot be without a chapter on scientific or empirical evidence. The seventh chapter provides an overview of the evidence for art therapy in personality disorders as it is presently available. My participation in the Dutch Trimbos Instituut's work group for the multidisciplinary guideline for the treatment of personality disorders, the care standard as representative of the arts therapies and my Ph.D. helped to bring about an intensive study of the literature.

Part II: The Workbook

I also developed a workbook and continually held it up to the scrutiny of reality and actual practice. The workbook offers a large number of assignments. They are described in practical terms and I hope they offer all art therapists' new ideas, show some familiar old ones in repackaged form and provide something to go on in devising new ones. These assignments have been collected for a number of years, and so it is not always clear exactly where they come from: some assignments have been around for a long time, some have been altered, and others I developed myself. I hope that this offers a rich collection for many art therapists to build on. It has certainly done so for me.

Part I

The Chapters

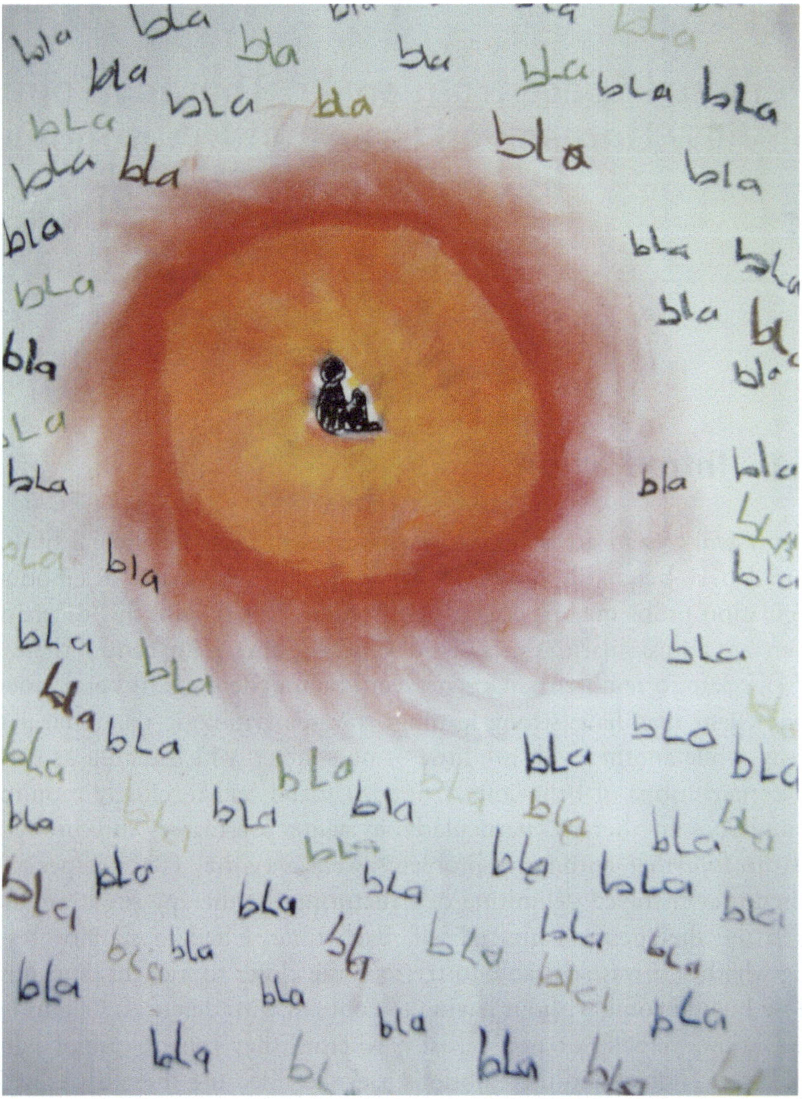

1

Personal Space from an Art Therapy Point of View Unresolved Issues with Autonomy as Central Factor

1.1 Introduction

In my work as an art therapist in a number of facets of mental health care, I have frequently dealt with clients with a wide range of emotion regulation problems or personality disorders. But despite this diversity, there are also similarities in a broad sense. Strikingly, the central themes often relate to remoteness-closeness and boundaries-lack of boundaries. One client may have strong leanings towards symbiotic relational patterns, while another will seek little or no contact, which manifests itself in certain forms of behaviour. I noticed that I had to closely monitor boundaries in therapy, particularly in acute psychiatry; this brought to the fore that autonomy problems were a central factor, especially when they involved delimiting or structuring the therapy situation and even the therapeutic contact itself. Each time, I had to start by testing whether it was advisable to try to come closer to a client, and how close I could come without having to contend with defences. Clients let you know, verbally or non-verbally, whether they can or cannot handle closer contact and the emotions it evokes. Because these issues with autonomy proved to be so central, I want to take a closer look at what

S. Haeyen, *Art Therapy and Emotion Regulation Problems*,
https://doi.org/10.1007/978-3-319-96773-8_1

might be termed the figurative personal space. This figurative space can be explored in art therapy: 'Man must again and again represent his inner reality in external form in order to progress..... (He) begins by experiencing his inward reality as something outside himself and he draws this reality back to himself in the course of integration. It is precisely this mechanism which enables man to progress beyond what he was' (Champernowne, 1968).

To my mind, this personal space is closely related to the concept of ego strength, to how the ego is structured and in how far it is developed. The self,[1] or the subjective, personal perception, is also of great importance. Self-determination can be recognised in a person's personal space. This personal space, which is often encountered in art therapy, thus becomes a symbol for the self-experience, for self-determination.

In discussing the development of this personal space, I will look briefly at ego development and the relationship between self and objects in the first years of life, linking this to the way a child's drawing develops. I will also consider the way the personal space is given shape in art therapy. In conclusion, I will discuss how art therapy can contribute to developing or rediscovering one's personal space.

1.2 The Phenomenon of Personal Space

Personal space is a rather vague concept often used figuratively but also literally in writing and speaking. In a figurative sense, it may refer to the position, the space you occupy as a person or the place a particular form of therapy occupies in the treatment team. In a literal sense, it may refer to the place you live, your crafts room or office or your retreat. Time and again, personal space proves to have a big influence on how you feel, on how you function. It then even seems to refer to something with substance.

---

[1]In this chapter, the self is regarded as part of the ego. The ego is the organiser that deals with the voice of conscience, aspirations and instincts and with the demands of the surroundings. The self refers to the way the individual sees himself or herself as a person, distinct from the objects in the external world. Succinctly, a person's individuality or uniqueness.

Viewed from how you experience it, having your own figurative personal space means you can rely on yourself, you have a sense of safety when alone and when in contact with others, and you have an integrated self-image. This includes experiencing your own boundaries, your ego's boundaries, defending them, and feeling that you are able to and have the courage to open the boundaries. This applies to contacts with others and to contacts you make with yourself, in which these different forces that put up and take down boundaries play an important role. This definition of personal space is very similar to the term 'ego strength' as it is used in psychological discourse.

1.3 Personal Space as Your Own Territory

1.3.1 Human Territory

In their Dutch-language book *Verboden toegang* (No Entry) from 1984, Bakker and Bakker-Rabdau write about the importance of having your own space, its function and behaviour in relation to it. The book is about human territory and mankind's territorial struggle. The subject and the way the authors treat it offer many tools for the practice of art therapy: for finding work methods and for acknowledging and understanding processes that take place in and around the personal space. Territoriality is a specific form of possessiveness or control. A person's territory consists of fields in which he or she has particular expertise, takes initiatives and bears responsibility—in other words, areas that are within his or her control. This refers to physical space and to aspects of our social and intellectual life.

People are faced with territorial conflicts on a daily basis. Territorial behaviour includes, for example, defining the area, setting up warning signs, defending the area tooth and nail, and perhaps making active attempts to expand it. *The core of every person's territory is the self, identity.* Autonomy, being autonomous, is having control, being in charge of yourself. The literal meaning of autonomous is self-regulating (Fig. 1.1).

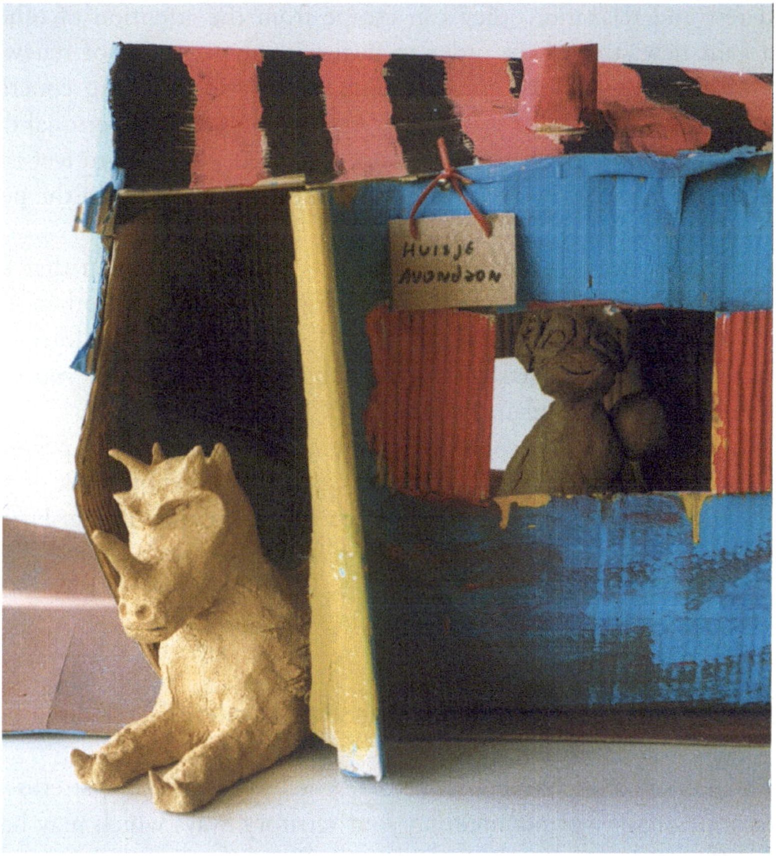

Fig. 1.1 John's personal space: the main character in his picture story lives in a hovel called Evening Sun Cottage, surrounded by a huge forest because, as John says, this person has a Homo sapiens phobia. His snarly, snappy hellhound protects him against all the aggressive people who come visiting

1.3.2 Several Territories: Function and Behaviour

A person's personal space consists of several different, individual territories. There is the private domain, which is the area a person demarcates to guarantee privacy. This aspect is so important for human beings that they will spend a great deal of time and energy defining and defending it. In addition, everyone needs a private space, a shelter. Here, people find rest and relaxation, they can escape from the attention of others and gain new strength in order to deal with the tensions of renewed interactions. This might mean reading a book or, in more concrete terms, having a studio or workplace. And there is also the personal distance: the literal and figurative distance you need if you are to feel safe, which is determined by your own confidence in yourself or in the people around you.

'The most unsettling symptom of being psychotic is often that the client has lost all sense of privacy. Thinking thoughts that others can read, your inner self being invaded by voices or other strange forces, so that you feel manipulated and are no longer in command of yourself' (Bakker & Bakker-Rabdau, 1984).

Where a number of people, and therefore also a number of personal territories, meet (e.g. in an art therapy group), we might speak of the *public arena*. Two types of territories can be distinguished here. Firstly, there is the psychological space, which refers to the psychological influence and the attention people give or receive in a group, and secondly, there is the action domain, the space where a person is active.

1.3.3 Territorial Behaviour and Personality Disorders

Personality disorders often involve learned or acquired patterns of behaviour or ways of maintaining your territory, ways which may have been efficient in the past but which now, in a different context, can no longer be considered adequate or healthy. People learn to respond in a way that reduces frustration. A person always chooses the response that has an effect. If, in the past, frustration or helplessness could be effectively met by an aggressive response, the person quickly learned to act aggressively. This response, which is controlled by an old 'form of adaptation stored away in the subconscious mind' (Molenaar, 2016), may not always be adequate in later situations.

Behavioural patterns relating to territoriality, in which aggressive conduct is extremely important, are largely based on individual experiences; they can be changed by new knowledge and new experiences, if a person feels sufficiently safe to be open to the possibility. Decisive factors in how people respond to an experience are their personal learning experience, their personal interpretation of the situation and the opportunities they have as a person have to control or defend their territory (a quick tongue, brute force). In the therapeutic situation, it is helpful to see what manners a person has found to deal with (or not to deal with) territorial problems.

1.4 Creating and Shaping the Personal Space

1.4.1 Ego Development and the Relationship Between the Self and the Objects

Your own territory, your personal space or your ego strength has its origins in ego development and the relationship between the self and the objects. In the early stages, it roughly boils down to this: there is no boundary between ego and non-ego. The distinction comes later. Boundaries arise between ego and non-ego and between good and bad. Ego functions develop rapidly and are practised with transitional objects and in the transitional area. Experiences are internalised. After this, children must find some way of defending or confirming their ego towards their surroundings. Integration takes places at around the age of three: a merging of positive and negative emotions for the object and integration of good and bad in the self, instead of splitting into a good and a bad self (Cullberg, 2003). If children form normal and safe attachments, they will develop their own self-awareness as well as sufficient independence. Attachment theory assumes that an unsafe and/or ambivalent attachment, which summons up feelings of anxiety and aggression, will result in a certain degree of ego weakness. A child's self-image and the relationships that develop are formed on the basis of the nature and quality of the attachment and detachment. As a result of ego weakness, stressful situations or other ordeals may lead to personality disorders, something that happens less readily in normal development.

1.4.2 Developments in a Child's Drawings and Formation of the Self

A form by which the self is frequently represented—often done by several clients independently of each other and usually without being asked to do so and—is the circle. We see all manner of variations, some of them subconscious and some consciously chosen. The circle also has an important role in the development of early childhood drawings (until around the age of four). A great deal has been written on the development of drawing and children's drawings. The circle has a special place in this regard. 'Ego awareness is documented in children's drawing by the circular form' (Strauss, 1986). The development of the circular form—through scribbles, tangles and complex spirals—goes hand in hand with the first experience of inner and outer. The child also develops the cross, which represents standing in the here and now.

'After the age of three, the circle and the cross merge into a single entity .... The circle, the centre of which is fixed by the point or the cross, describes the life situation at this age. In such a drawing, children represent their relationship to inner and outer, and the point or the intersection stands for themselves and inner space. With these signs, children illustrate for the first time how they experience themselves and their surroundings. The point and the cross are inside the circle and represent the "I-form"' (Strauss, 1986, p. 29). First, the lines of the cross or star radiate from a central point to the circumference of the circle, staying within the boundaries, but later they extend beyond and into the child's environment.

This development in children's drawings corresponds to the first period of personality development discussed earlier in this chapter. There we also saw that many of the disorders for which clients seek psychiatric help have their origins in early childhood. These aspects in particular make it so interesting that in the drawings of adult clients, the circle is also often used as an I-form with a certain boundary between inner and outer, representing how their inner space looks. The circle, a universal symbol, here symbolises the self.

During the drawing process, the circle can evoke very divergent associations such as safety and security, but also coercion and oppression. Later forms of expressing the self in visual terms are the human form, the 'tree person', the tree and the house as enclosure. Other abstract forms may have this function as well. They are forms that have been drawn on the basis of an inner perception. Colours, lines, shapes and use of materials play an important role in bringing to expression the emotional significance, both in the circle and in the later expressive forms (on this, see also the annex entitled 'What makes the expressive medium so powerful') (Figs. 1.2 and 1.3).

A few examples from the art work of a number of clients:

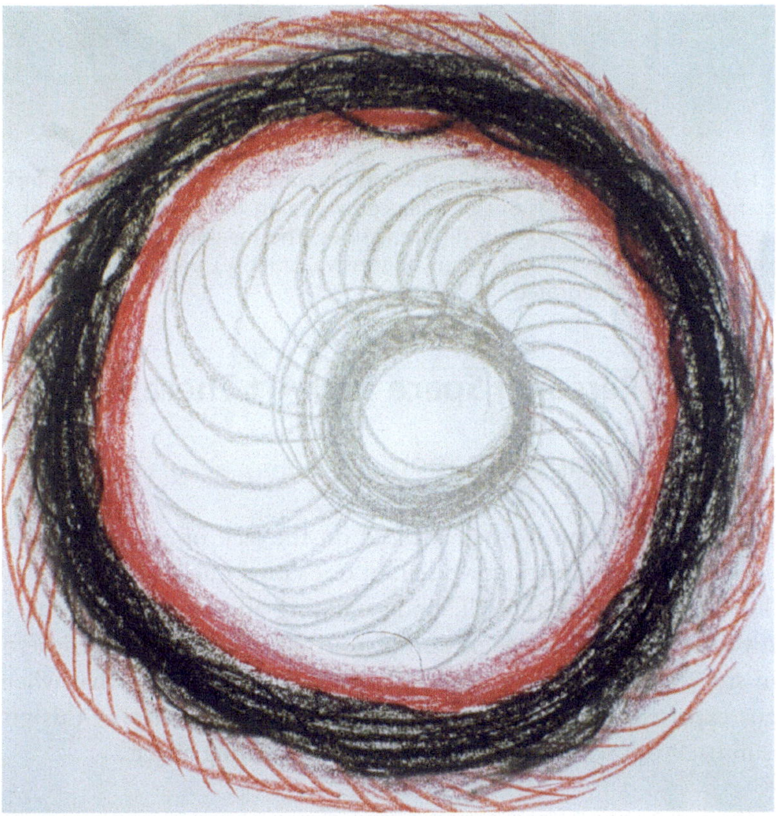

Fig. 1.2 Strong defences/strong boundaries

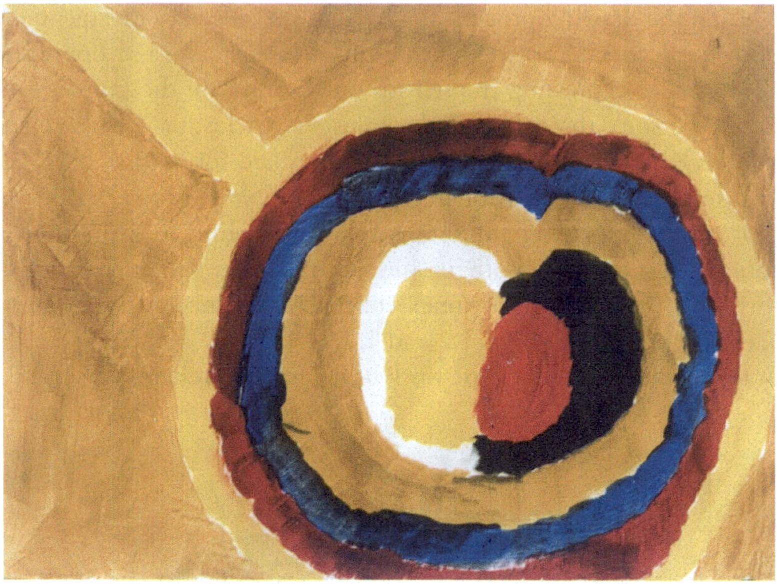

Fig. 1.3 On his own initiative, client Kevin portrays 'his inner self'. He compensates for the fact that it is out of balance by adding the line to the corner. His inner self is split into two very different sides (the meaning he gives this portrayal: peaceful, good mood versus aggressive, sombre) and the impression it makes is far from integrated

1.5 The Personal Space and Art Therapy

1.5.1 The Therapy Situation

The therapy situation is often focused on the lack of ego development or lack of awareness of the own self, of one's own nucleus and one's own actions. Experiencing the self, understanding and appreciating the self and your own actions, recognition of yourself and your experience/your own story is an important object of therapy. I have found that when a client experiences that first fundamental step on the way to this goal, this in itself can restore the balance or have a healing effect.

1.5.2 Aspects of Working in Art Therapy Relating to the Personal Space

When clients make an art work, autonomy issues immediately come up. Making something, particularly something of your own, from within, is an act of autonomy over which you have control. While you are working on it, you can also be in touch with your inner feelings, your motivation. This is how art therapy can play an important role in helping clients to regain a certain autonomy and, more in general, in an ego-strengthening treatment process.

In the most extreme sense, art therapy in itself—showing something of yourself or perhaps a figurative representation—can result in alienation from the self. This can happen when all contact with the self, with the other or with the surroundings is frightening and must be avoided to maintain a sense of self-preservation. An example of this is the client who painted a few coloured areas. At my request, she added something figurative and felt that she was immediately alienated from her painting. She could not make a link of any kind between the tree she had produced and herself. Even abstract, schematic or stereotypical designs can sometimes mean self-preservation or avoidance of contact, and this can serve to reduce anxiety.

Clients can come in contact with their own feelings by making a creative work. 'A person will first have to be in contact with what belongs to him or her before attempting a contact with anything else' (Molenaar, 1992/2016). Coming in contact with what is uniquely yours takes place through self-observation but also through observation of the things around you (perhaps things you made, shapes and nature) or through symbols. Experiencing boundaries and maintaining contact with yourself in relation to others have its place, alongside making contact with others and sharing experiences. Particularly in art therapy, this is one of the most important background reasons to work with creative arts. Essential aspects are, for example, how large or small your space on the shared paper is, how you fill this space, the similarities and differences between the various group members, how you work together, or what you said or did not say.

1.5.3 The Role of the Art Therapist

As an art therapist, I respond to the given situation by the way I use the medium: the choice of materials, the degree of structure and the nature of the assignment or approach. I try to make this fit in with what the client has said or can cope with. It is important that in my attitude as a therapist, I make sure that the situation is safe enough, that I structure it, but more importantly, that I make myself very clear. A person will first have to experience some degree of safety or trust before even contemplating a focus on contact with him or herself, or with the own uniqueness. Particularly if there are difficulties with autonomy, it is important to respect the space that the client apparently needs and to be cautious with the interventions you use. In such cases, based on the client's experience, interventions can readily be perceived as demanding, accusing, intrusive or even taking away control. The client can exhibit anxious behaviour or do what he thinks is expected of him; the situation can become unsafe and threatening and because of the anxiety this arouses, perhaps even alienating.

1.5.4 Regaining Personal Space in Its Most Basic Form: Psychotic Disintegration

Clients with personality disorders sometimes also have a psychotic or dissociative disorder on Axis I. A psychosis can take on various forms; it may involve decompensation, falling to pieces, but may also involve delusions. During a delusion, images arise that are related but that have an unreal, delusional meaning for their maker. In art therapy, an answer to this is working in accordance with reality or focusing on reality—for example, the reality of the materials used. A client experiencing psychotic disintegration is not able to create a coherent picture; he has a hard time imposing boundaries, and there seems to be little distinction between inner and outer. This is sometimes expressed in an art work in which the various elements seem to be totally unrelated or disordered, sometimes in art work which exhibits very little differentiation. In such a case, it is important, first and foremost, to arrive at some form of integration—in other words, coherence. The client needs to be able to regain a small piece of her territory, her personal space. This starts by overcoming chaos.

It takes place partly through the process of making an art work, since this is a process that requires ordering and organising. This aspect is about how a client struggles with the art materials and conquers the form. Chaos in an art work can be countered by adding aspects such as directions, contour, frameworks, symmetry and so on (Beljon, 2011). Form can be regarded as order in chaos (Molenaar, 2016). In working creatively, a basic quality, in particular for clients with psychotic symptoms, is being able to regain control by ordering, designing, structuring, exerting influence and determining.

In addition to this side of art work, there is the expressive side. Working on the basis of the expressive side in art therapy means: 'Expressing emotions in the form of art works through creative mediums in a psychotherapeutic framework where the client, on a largely subconscious level, uses materials such as paint, chalk and clay to restore his intrapsychic relations' (Wertheim-Cahen, 1991). For clients with psychotic symptoms, another equally basic quality of making art works is seeing something of themselves in the work itself (forms, lines, colours and themes), something of their own world of experience (expression) and contact with their own feelings while making the works (Figs. 1.4 and 1.5).

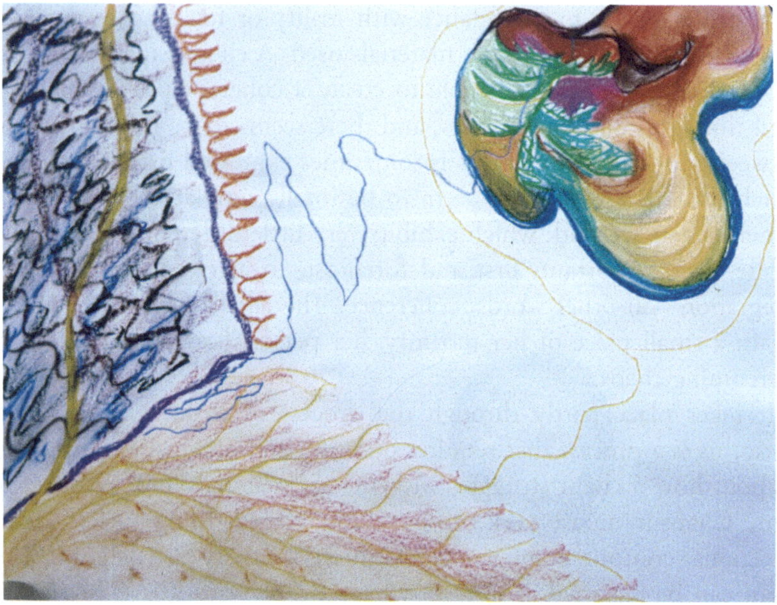

Fig. 1.4 Work made by two clients working together: each in their own personal space, making contact with the other on paper

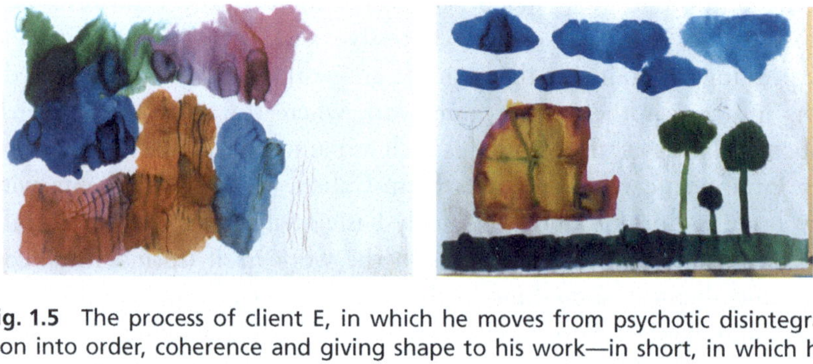

Fig. 1.5 The process of client E, in which he moves from psychotic disintegration into order, coherence and giving shape to his work—in short, in which he conquers chaos

Giving shape to a work can symbolise or represent experiences, wishes, emotions or thoughts. A link can be made between the work produced and the experience, between the person and the disorder. The degree of structure and the manner in which I create structure for clients with psychotic disintegration largely depends on the person. Offering too much structure deprives people of the opportunity to take greater control themselves, to conquer chaos. The client's anxiety level is always the determining factor.

1.5.5 Regaining and Giving Shape to the Personal Space in Personality Disorders

The aspects of making an art work as described above are also important in regaining one's own territory, regaining control, autonomy as well as self-esteem and self-confidence. In personality disorders in which the psychotic disintegration has abated, is less present or is simply not in the picture, these are important aspects as well, but they are at a different level. For instance, a client can regain control by making a complex abstract form. Then, the dominant aspect is not fighting against chaos, but learning to control it.

On the expressive side, art therapy is about:

- giving concrete shape to your personal space, to the self or self-image in any form
- giving shape to your own story
- giving free rein to emotions and representing emotions
- finding your own characteristic form in which to work
- making contact with the side of yourself that you usually have less contact with (in an inner conflict).

Just which goal is targeted during therapy, and so which aspect (control or expression) will receive more emphasis, depends on what, in your estimation, a person needs to change so as not to become deadlocked again, and how attainable the objective is, measured against the personal capabilities of the client at this point in time. Sometimes, your estimation will be that a person needs to change more than is viable right now; this is a problem the entire treatment team will need to address.

1.5.6 Benefits of Art Therapy

As has been described, in a therapeutic situation, art therapy has a number of possible benefits compared to other forms of therapy. Its inherently creative nature, the fact that clients produce a concrete piece of work, gives it ego-strengthening qualities thanks to the fact that clients see a part of themselves in their work. It allows clients to look at themselves and their own product from a distance and to respond to it. And they get a response—feedback—from others. The active behaviour involved in creating an art work yields a direct experience, and the materials used invite clients to respond physically and emotionally. Creating an art work can be revealing because images sometimes emerge unexpectedly or unintentionally; this may lead to a reduced sense of control. And it offers a relatively safe situation because not only can it be revealing, it can also be concealing. Clients may perhaps regard the substance of a work they make as something that is not part of them (but perhaps will be at a later stage) as simply 'make-believe' and 'whatever came to mind'.

It often involves experiences that a person has stored away and that are difficult to express in words—for example, because the roots of the disorder lie in the preverbal phase of development, or because, when the person had this experience, it was too huge, too traumatic, and may have made the client literally 'the prisoner of his images' (Wertheim-Cahen, 1991). Creating a piece of work and discussing the creative aspects can sometimes serve as a link or an entrance to such experiences better than words can do (Fig. 1.6).

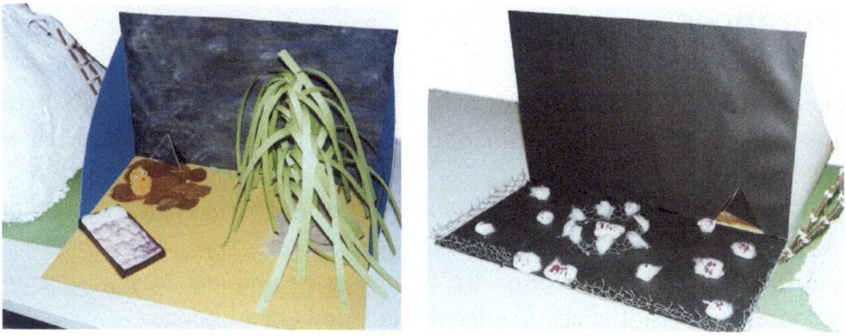

Fig. 1.6 The beginning of the process of giving shape to client Jennifer's personal space, from the safe place dominated by regression (left) to its dark side: the place of self-harm, isolation and corresponding emotions (right). The door between this place and the first place gives her a certain sense of safety

1.6 Summary

This chapter describes the phenomenon of personal space and how this is a basic theme in art therapy for clients with personality disorders. Personal space is closely related to the concept of ego strength, to how the ego is structured and in how far it is developed. We have looked at the relationship between personality development in early childhood and at how children's drawings develop; we have looked at giving shape to works in art therapy made by adult clients with personality disorders. Art therapy can strengthen the client's autonomy and improve ego strength. Shaping one's personal space (depending on the person and his or her personal issues) can take place at various levels: from conscious to subconscious, from overcoming chaos and regaining control to being emotionally involved in giving shape to your own personal space. Art therapy may initiate a process towards developing, investigating, recognising and expanding your personal space.

References

Bakker, C. B., & Bakker-Rabdau, M. K. (1984). *Verboden toegang* [No trespassing! Explorations in human territoriality]. Antwerpen: Nederlansde boekhandel.

Beljon, J. J. (2011). *Zo doe je dat; grondbeginselen van vormgeving*. Amsterdam: Arbeiderspers.

Champernowne, H. I. (1968). *Art therapy as an adjunct to psychotherapy*. Lecture at the Art Therapy Conference at Cumberland Lodge.

Cullberg, J. (2003). *Moderne psychiatrie*. Amsterdam: Ambo/Anthos.

Molenaar, E. (1992). Het weten van de handen. *Tijdschrift voor Creatieve Therapie*, 1992–1.

Molenaar, E. (2016). *Beeldwaarneming; begrippenapparaat bij een benoemingssysteem voor beeldend werk*. Venray: Multicopy-Venray-Venlo-Parkstad.

Strauss, M. (1986). *Kindertekeningen*. Zeist: Christofoor.

Wertheim-Cahen, T. (1991). *Getekend Bestaan*. Utrecht: Stichting ICODO.

2

Client with a Diagnosis of a Borderline Personality Disorder: Responsible and Competent!? Art Therapy and Severe Cluster B Personality Disorders

Working with clients diagnosed as having severe cluster B personality disorders, also known as lower level borderline psychopathology, gives rise to considerable difficulties in therapeutic practice. In this chapter, I offer a framework and explain how this can be applied to art therapy. To begin, let us consider a specific case.

Case: Maria

Maria is a young woman with a severe cluster B personality disorder. She already has considerable experience with treatment and therapy. She has previously been admitted to a clinic for personality disorders but could not handle this. The admission was too intensive, as indicated by an increased incidence of acting out behaviour. Maria currently has two forms of outpatient therapy: talk therapy and art therapy. The talk therapy, which takes place once every two to three weeks, is aimed at improving the balance between burden and coping capacity. The aim of the art therapy, which is offered once a week, is to expand the client's grip on her life and her capacity to cope. When the tension becomes too great for Maria, she can make use of a time-out arrangement entailing admission to a clinic for one or two days.

S. Haeyen, *Art Therapy and Emotion Regulation Problems*,
https://doi.org/10.1007/978-3-319-96773-8_2

During our initial contact, Maria tells me that she really does not know what to do with art therapy. She nevertheless decides to try it. Maria only makes very limited eye contact. She prefers to keep both her interpersonal contact and what she depicts during therapy at a very safe distance. She opts for familiar work methods. She chooses to paint wet-on-wet, for example, which she is familiar with from the Steiner school.

Her painting gradually takes on more personal meaning, which she is also able to express in words. Some trust and sense of security have thus developed.

Maria also wants to work with clay, which is familiar to her as well. While doing this, she talks about her boyfriend and her father—relationships with which she is preoccupied. She doesn't know how she should view these relationships and is not happy with how they are going. I ask her to form a human figure, out of clay, to represent herself. After she has done this, I ask her to form a second human figure. When she is done, I ask her to position the figures with respect to each other in a manner which she sees as fitting (see Fig. 2.1). She positions herself sitting with short, limp arms in a reclining posture which looks to me like it cannot possibly be held without help. Maria sees this as well. She tells me that the other person is a man. This figure is given a sturdy stance. Maria spends time searching for a good way to position the two figures. She views her own clay figure as dependent and passive; she views the other figure as independent and strong. She says that she hates feeling dependent and does not want the man to offer her support by standing either behind her or next to her. She does not want this, so how should she arrange the figures then? At a great distance from each other? No, that's too much distance. What to do about the reclining posture of her clay figure then? It cannot stand alone. She finally comes up with a solution: she gives 'herself' a nice, purple, velvet ball to hold against her belly. Doing this optically brings her figure into balance! According to Maria, the purple ball symbolises caring better for herself than she normally does. The ball feels nice and soft and brings her more into equilibrium. By giving her clay figure the ball, Maria pays attention to herself instead of waiting for someone else to help her or think something up.

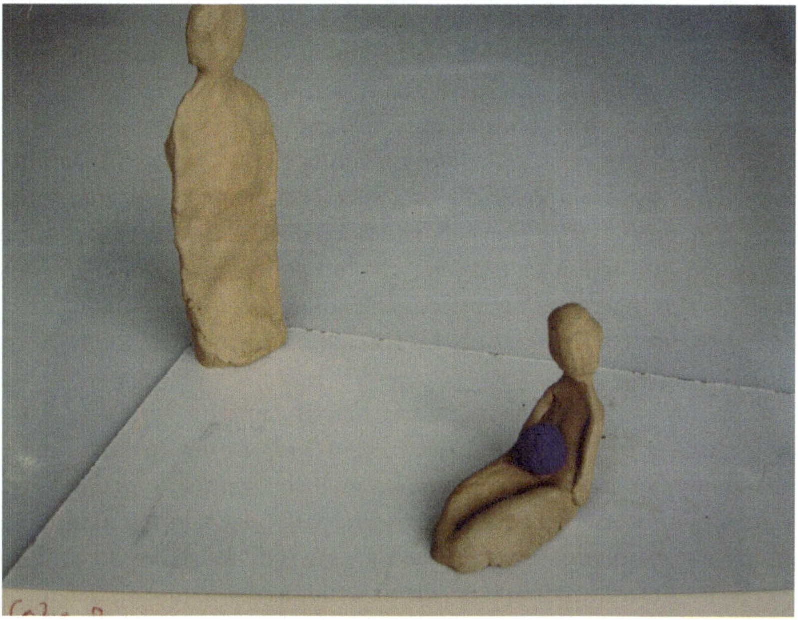

Fig. 2.1 Two figures in clay, the purple ball as a symbol for caring for herself

During the next session, Maria says that she found herself thinking a lot about that session. It was the first time that she 'actually benefited from art therapy'. But before we proceed further, she wants to talk about something. She still dreads coming so much. And she does not know if she wants to keep coming; maybe she should just stop therapy.

2.1 What Is Actually Happening?

Splitting or what is often referred to as black-and-white, all-or-nothing thinking has now occurred. The inner conflict between 'it did me good' and 'I don't want this confrontation' has been projected directly into the therapeutic relationship. Rather than go along with this by trying to convince Maria of the usefulness of the therapy, the therapist must stand aside but also remain involved at the same time. Maria does not connect the two experiences and has a strong tendency to react impulsively.

As an alternative, the therapist can appeal to Maria's autonomy. 'I understand what is happening. What do you think a solution might be?' You then ignore destructive solutions until something positive presents itself; at the same time, it is important to establish limits. Reflecting on what took place and on limits can be quite stimulating. I asked Maria, for example, if the previous session had made such a deep impression on her that she had felt a need for destructive behaviour such as self-mutilation or excessive alcohol consumption. Her response was that this had not happened and that she was not completely undone by what had taken place. This rational approach thus allowed Maria to relativise a bit.

While talking about things, Maria herself came up with the idea of doing nothing further during the current session, but to take time to think about things and then let me know if she wanted to proceed with the therapy or not. This was a good idea, particularly in the light of the importance of maintaining autonomy and individual responsibility. I nevertheless introduced an element of structure by requiring her to call with her decision at an agreed upon time. One week later, she called with the announcement that she wanted to continue after all.

2.2 What Is a Severe Cluster B Personality Disorder?

A personality disorder is a particular style of interpersonal and more general behaviour showing a stable but dysfunctional pattern. This pattern involves old behaviour which has become anchored in the person's development and thus is a part of the individual's personality.

The DSM 5 (American Psychiatric Association, 2013/2014) speaks in the case of borderline personality disorder of a 'pervasive pattern of instability of interpersonal relationships, self-image, and affects, with marked impulsivity beginning by early adulthood and present in a variety of contexts'. In short: instability of thinking, feeling and acting. Impulsivity, mood swings and thinking which is all-or-nothing are among the characteristics that stand out most for this client group.

Also characteristic of the disorder is that the anxiety experienced by the person does not manifest itself completely: it is too great for this. What is more, the person does not consider the anxiety part of his or her own self, but projects it into the relationship and the ongoing interaction instead. With the group of clients classified as cluster B, very weak identity formation is also presumed to be the case (Eurelings-Bontekoe, Verheul, & Snellen, 2009; Ingenhoven, van Reekum, van Luyn, & Luyten, 2012; Linehan, 1993). A stable self-image and sense of self have not emerged during the person's development. When a person does not have a stable self-image and, related to this, a stable image of others, perceptions of the boundaries between the sense of self and others can become blurred. The boundaries are continually perceived differently, depending on the situation and the people interacting. As mentioned, what the person with a borderline personality disorder then experiences is not felt but projected into the ongoing interaction. The context thus determines their behaviour.

People diagnosed with a borderline or severe cluster B personality disorder are also known to constantly try to find security in the company of someone they have idealised. But because their own identity is so diffuse or weak, the proximity of an idealised other can simultaneously elicit the fear of losing oneself in the contact and thus lead to distancing from the idealised other at the same time. Distancing oneself too much from others can, in turn, elicit the fear of disappearing all together. One can thus speak of separation anxiety or a fear of abandonment and merger anxiety or a fear of intimacy. Attraction and rejection, separation anxiety and merger anxiety, all of these mechanisms operate quite strongly due to the combination of the aforementioned factors in clients with a borderline personality disorder.

Other common symptoms are self-mutilation and acute psychotic or dissociation episodes. For the lower level group, the symptoms can be quite severe: contact can hardly be tolerated. For this reason, monitoring the closeness and distance during the therapeutic contact is of critical importance, as is maintaining at least a minimum of contact in the working relationship.

2.3 Important Assumptions for Treatment of a Severe Cluster B Personality Disorder

A source of inspiration for the treatment of clients with a severe cluster B personality disorder is the theory of Dawson and MacMillan (1993). According to these authors, the traditional role of the empathic care provider is one that only reinforces the idea of the client with a borderline disorder as incompetent, out of control and incapable of taking responsibility for himself or herself. As a result, a pathological relational pattern is simply repeated and maintained. For Dawson and MacMillan, the most important assumption for treatment is that the client is a responsible and competent adult. Autonomy must thus stand central; hospitalisation should be avoided or discouraged. The care provider is involved but neutral and only imposes limits on what is to be tolerated by himself or herself and the institution.

The object of art therapy for clients with a severe cluster B personality disorder is to teach them to give direction to their lives and expand their coping capacities within the limits and the possibilities they have.

2.4 Art Therapy for People Diagnosed with a Borderline Personality Disorder

Art therapy offers expression but also numerous structuring possibilities which fit nicely with the specific themes to be addressed during the treatment of a client with a borderline personality disorder—emotion regulation and impulse regulation, for example. Art therapy involves acting and experiencing, raising awareness, giving expression and making visible but also the possibility of remaining hidden and only going halfway. These characteristics mean that control over expression and action can be experienced and practised within the therapeutic context. Clients with a borderline disorder often have a diffuse and negative image of themselves, and they often get caught up in intense emotions which directly elicit a given cognitive or behavioural reaction on their part. Giving form to one's emotions and the content of one's thoughts calls for a structuring of experience and thought. And art therapy can help with this process.

Reflection occurs within art therapy on a number of levels and with respect to a variety of processes: the direct act of creating something, the content of the creation, the experience of creating something, thoughts regarding what has been created and social functioning when it comes to showing and discussing what has been created. Clients with a borderline personality disorder, however, often proceed directly from feeling to acting and they are often completely controlled by negative thoughts about their actions. The integration of feelings, thinking and acting is therefore an important objective of treatment for a borderline disorder. And to frame therapeutic experiences and promote integration, it is important that communication also takes place and words are given to the experiences gathered during art therapy.

2.5 Objectives of Art Therapy for This Group

The general objectives which can be outlined for art therapy and the contact with an art therapist are as follows for clients with severe borderline personality disorder:

- Processing emotions
- Imposing structure
- Handling conflict
- Strengthening ego
- Improving social functioning
- Expanding behavioural repertoire

While working with this target group, all these objectives will be addressed at some point. Critical for working effectively with clients diagnosed as having a severe cluster B personality disorder is monitoring the distance and closeness of the contact and the medium being used during a therapy session. Of particular importance is establishing the right tone to start with. The contact can quickly get too close for the client or remain too great at a distance. As the therapist, you must strive to stay in the area in between. Given that the target group involves individuals for whom contact is unstable and impulsivity is characteristic, it is important for you to offer absolute clarity with regard to any agreements made and the therapeutic stance taken. In this way, the client and therapist jointly determine the therapeutic context.

Just how I work with this target group and how the aforementioned objectives enter into the therapy will be illustrated in the following sections. This will be done in terms of specific aspects of art therapy and just how these get translated for use with this particular target group.

2.6 Specific Aspects of Art Therapy and Their Translation for Use with the Target Group

Act rather than talk. Other disciplines tend to think that language and talk play no role in non-verbal therapies. This is simply not true. Language is an important component of the therapeutic art, as language is used to attach words to experiences, label emotions and differentiate between various aspects of experience. Acting nevertheless stands central in art therapy, as this offers a very different starting point than talking.

Connect verbal and non-verbal. The questions to ask yourself as an art therapist are: Do the product of the work and the work process itself show a relationship to what is said? Is the explanation provided for a work in keeping with what it shows? This target group often tends to separate these aspects, leaving little or no correspondence between them. For instance, the client can work intensely on something but later say that its production was 'nothing special… who needs art therapy anyway?' Conversely, an entire story may be told about a given product while it actually shows very little (does not reflect what is described in the story) or shows something quite different.

Make sure that feeling, seeing, thinking and acting are all concretely and perceptibly included. For someone with a cluster B personality disorder, seeing and feeling are often directly connected to acting. Thinking and distancing rarely occur together. During treatment, including art therapy, you try to influence this impulsive behaviour by introducing thinking between feeling and acting. You work to let rational thinking take the lead rather than feeling. Emotions can, after all, say one thing on one occasion and something else on another, and this can be very confusing and exhausting.

In art therapy, materials are also placed between feeling and acting to slow the intervening steps and make them more apparent. You handle and feel the materials; a particular medium or theme allows you to feel certain things, act in a certain manner, see what happens once you act in a certain manner and think about what has happened and what is called up in you after acting in a certain manner; then you think some more, and during the follow-up discussion you see, think, feel and act. Did you distance yourself or stay very close to what you made? Are you proud of what you made or not? During most interpersonal and verbal interactions, all these processes unfold much more quickly, making it difficult to identify them and view them separately (Fig. 2.2).

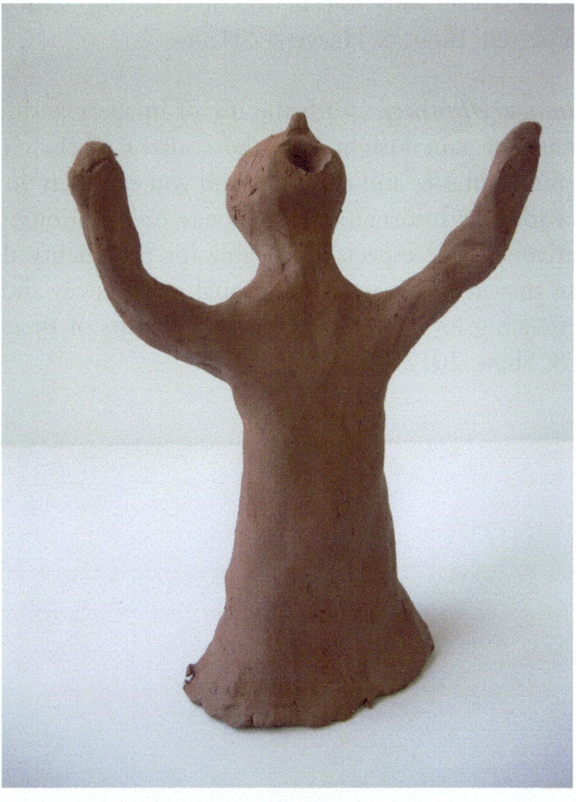

Fig. 2.2 Schema of abandonment or dependency

Connect to preverbal processes/basic schemas. In thinking about oneself, basic schemas exist such as 'I'm worthless' and so 'my work is worthless'. These basic schemas generally emerge at a young age and have sometimes from before the development of language. These often unconscious patterns of thought are rooted in the individual.

In cases of sexual abuse (this group frequently exhibits traumas), the basic schema can, for example, be 'people just mess with me' or 'I'm simply an object'. This was certainly the case at the time of the trauma. So it is important that the autonomy of the individual is emphasised and placed central during therapy. The client determines the course of things; the client can and may influence things. This also means that you, as the therapist, do not impose a particular medium or method but, rather, consult with the client on the medium and methods to be used. As the therapist, your role is one of coaching, structuring (Van Vreeswijk, Broersen, Bloo, & Haeyen, 2012).

Call upon imagery/fantasy. With the use of imagery and fantasy, you and the client can gain insight into the content of their experiential world, thoughts, fantasies and demons. And you can then do something therapeutic with this information The focus on emotions (positive as well as negative) can be especially suitable for personality disorder clients, because they tend to avoid emotional experiences and may have missed experiencing joy and play as key ingredients of their childhood (Lockwood & Shaw, 2012) (Fig. 2.3).

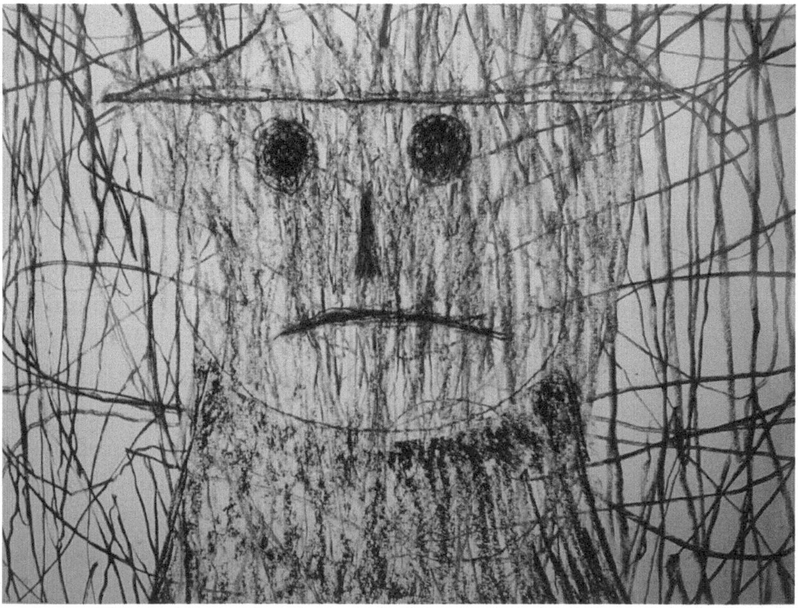

Fig. 2.3 During an art therapy activity, Marjorie comes into contact with an imaginary fear which repeatedly occurs when things are not going well with her. A black man wearing a cape is following her, which gives her an anxious, tense feeling. She knows he is not real but she still can't rid herself of him and the feeling emanated by his presence. Marjorie arrived at the session in a very emotionally charged state. Because of her anxiety, which also manifested itself in her art therapy activity, she initially wanted to escape—her drawing movements literally went off the edges of the paper. When asked to give form to what she was experiencing, a portrait of a black man emerged. While looking at it, she said 'Now I can at least look him in the eye'. By giving her fantasy concrete form, Marjorie no longer felt so anxious. She clearly felt more in control of things because she was now able to look at things within a clearly delimited and tangible situation

Materials speak to your feelings, your emotions and your senses. In working with this target group, the therapist must be aware of the influence of the material selected to work with. Providing materials (or not providing them) and the manner of working must be carefully attuned to this influence. Attention to sufficient structure is also important. Individuals with severe borderline personality problems are easily overwhelmed, which means that what they experience during therapy can quickly become too much. The tendency to distance oneself, for example, by breaking off treatment can then increase greatly. It is definitely a contraindication for this form of therapy if clients are so overwhelmed by what they experience that the therapy is no longer productive. Their anxiety becomes too great, and a good working relationship with the therapist cannot be established.

For clients with a borderline personality disorder, there is the additional danger of disintegration. Psychotic or dissociative symptoms can be elicited by overly intense experiences or memories. In particular, working with clay can have this effect because the material is so formless and is known to make a strong appeal to emotions. Just how, when and with what degree of structure the use of clay is introduced should therefore be carefully thought through. Working with clay is not without some risk and requires knowledge and experience.

Art therapy can partially counter the need for acting out, self-mutilation, substance abuse and thrill-seeking. Clients in art therapy can rid themselves of tension and start to feel themselves again, but now productively instead of destructively. Depictions of cutting, scratching and other aggressive themes can work constructively during art therapy by bringing dangerous matters to the fore without them actually taking place. In the process itself and in the later discussion, attention should focus on these themes (cutting, other aggression) and not on working through in an explorative sense. In other words: What have you just done? How do you think it looks? What does it tell you? How are you going to handle this?

Introduce structure via materials and methods. It is important, as already mentioned, to introduce structure via the materials and methods selected for use, but also to keep the client's need for autonomy in mind when doing this. You offer a safe and secure environment with perhaps some additional support, but no more than this. Responsibility must be kept with the client.

There is usually a clear need on the part of the client for some structure. Providing a pencil and ruler and asking the client to work with them in a particular manner does provide strong support. However, when carrying this out, chances are that clients will not feel a connection with what they have been asked to do, and disinterest or anxiety may be the result. Frustration and anxiety can quickly give rise to problems in the contact with the client and even result in a complete lack of contact. The contact which has been established with a client is generally quite fragile and must therefore be carefully monitored. In other words, remember: consult with clients rather than dictating what they should do, but do provide some structure.

Focus on the here and now. By focusing on the here and now, you are in a position to address just how the client handles all aspects of the visual art process and his or her contact with others. The primary concern is the experience of the moment.

Use the medium to minimise the possibility of transference. Art therapy limits the potential for transference between client and therapist, and so it can literally be placed between the two of you if the contact quickly becomes charged or confusing and unclear. In art therapy, the famous triangular relationship of client—medium—therapist is always present. And this is a welcome aspect. The contact between client and therapist is less cluttered and more manageable in art therapy, making it more productive. The chances of the interpersonal contact becoming too close are limited by ensuring that clients focus on themselves.

2.7 The Art Work Produced and Its Functions When Working with This Target Group

Characteristic of art therapy in contrast to other forms of creative therapy is that a tangible product is generated. And this product has a number of other important features (Meijer-Degen, 1994; Schweizer et al., 2009).

Clearly visible. The product generated during art therapy is not fleeting and therefore often more controllable than other creative therapeutic outcomes.

Can be viewed from a distance. Both literally and figuratively, the work can be viewed from a distance. One can literally take a few steps back but also figuratively take some distance to view a piece. Follow-up commentary and the assignment of a title but also other forms of self-reflection invite the client to think. This is of particular importance for this target group because such thinking and reflection can expand their emotional and behavioural control.

Distance can also promote reality testing. What is perceived? Was this the intention? Is the description of what is depicted accurate? Sometimes even describing what is being viewed can be quite difficult for this target group.

Can serve different functions. In art therapy, matters can be given concrete form, significance can be attached to these forms, and as a result, important matters acknowledged and perhaps even dealt with. Clients can indulge their fantasies in what they have made and may choose to take care of it or watch over it. The product can thus be treated as a good luck charm (talisman) or a scapegoat.

Continues to exist, shows continuity. By continuing to exist, the art product can counter impulsivity. An evaluation of the works produced during a certain period is a lesson in experiencing continuity, in contrast to only feeling the tension of that day. It can counter splitting or, in the other words, the occurrence of black-and-white, all-or-nothing thinking, as in the case of Maria: coming to the therapy today was very difficult and confrontational for her, but at the same time, she viewed her creation of a work at the previous session as part of a very positive experience. It was stored in her memory in the form of the art work.

Both concealing and revealing. Clients can hide behind a work or, in other words, express something without sharing directly. They can also make themselves visible via their work.

Provides a mirror. The products of art therapy allow clients to look at themselves, at their own way of doing things, and to examine the content of their thoughts. The products can confront, reinforce or shed new light on matters. They can form a bridge between the internal and the external or the past, the present and the future. And they make the occurrence of splitting in the experiential world of the client explicit and visible (Fig. 2.4).

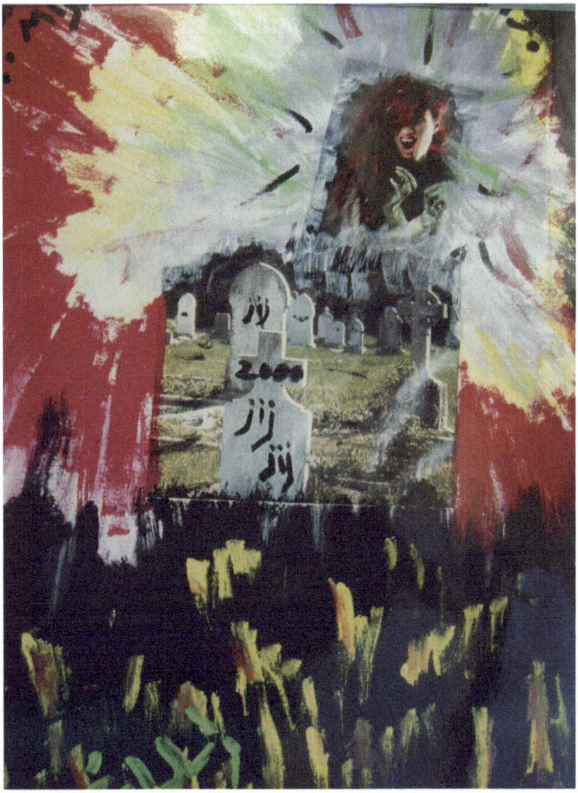

Fig. 2.4 Marlene sometimes produces very controlled, sweet, little pieces of work in pastel colours showing 'bears and flowers' even though she mainly uses her art therapy to create and project herself into large, dark, intense, expressive works with 'revenge' as their theme. She is both of these but, for her, they appear to be two unrelated parts of her, which she finds difficult. The negative themes which manifest themselves in her works are very characteristic for the target group described here: self-mutilation, impulsive expression, anger/rage, thoughts of suicide and the question 'Who am I?'

2.8 In Conclusion

The process of working towards greater integration, as described above, is a process which takes a considerable amount of time. Time is also what working with this target group demands of the therapist. The manner of working described here and the factors which are known to be operative in art therapy nevertheless elicit, in my experience, clearly positive results for both the client and therapist. Experience has shown that this manner of conducting art therapy reduces acting out, reduces problematic client/therapist relationships and helps prevent regression. Clients learn to take responsibility for their own behaviour and feel competent enough to regulate their emotions. The care provider gets less entangled in the therapeutic interaction than with other forms of therapy. I notice that, as an art therapist, I have a clear advantage over other therapists because I can call in art mediums and put them to use as I deem necessary and best. This makes the therapeutic relationship with clients suffering from severe borderline personality issues more straightforward and manageable, which obviously helps them and does justice to the objectives which they have set for themselves.

2.9 Summary

In this chapter, art therapy with clients diagnosed as having a severe cluster B personality disorder is described and linked to Dawson and MacMillan's relationship management theory. The important qualities of art therapy but also critical aspects of the medium and methods are translated for use with this specific target group.

References

American Psychiatric Association. (2013). *Diagnostic and statistical manual of mental disorders* (5th ed.). Washington, DC: Author.

American Psychiatric Association. (2014). *Handboek voor de classificatie van psychische stoornissen (DSM-5)* [Diagnostic and statistical manual of mental disorders] (5th ed.) (M. W. Hengeveld, Supervision Trans.). Amsterdam: Boom.

Dawson, D., & MacMillan, H. L. (1993). *Relationship management of the borderline patient; from understanding to treatment.* New York: Brunner/Mazel Publishers.

Eurelings-Bontekoe, E. H. M., Verheul, R., & Snellen, W. M. (Eds.) (2009). *Handboek persoonlijkheidspathologie* [Handbook on personality pathology] (2nd ed.). Houten: Bohn Stafleu van Loghum.

Ingenhoven, T., van Reekum, M., van Luyn, B., & Luyten, P. (Eds.) (2012). *Handboek borderline persoonlijkheidsstoornis* [Handbook on borderline personality disorder]. Utrecht: De Tijdstroom.

Linehan, M. M. (1993). *Cognitive-behavioural treatment of borderline personality disorder.* New York, NY: Guildford Press.

Lockwood, G., & Shaw, I. A. (2012). Schema therapy and the role of joy and play. In M. van Vreeswijk, J. Broersen, & M. Nadort (Eds.), *The Wiley-Blackwell handbook of schema therapy* (pp. 209–228). New York, NY: Wiley.

Meijer-Degen, F. (1994). Partners in therapie. *Tijdschrift voor creatieve therapie, 3*, 70–76.

Schweizer, C., Bruyn, J., Haeyen, S., Henskens, B., Rutten-Saris, M., & Visser, H. (2009). *Handboek beeldende therapie: Uit de verf* [Handbook of art therapy: Express yourself]. Houten: Bohn Stafleu van Loghum.

Van Vreeswijk, M., Broersen, J., Bloo, J., & Haeyen, S. (2012). Techniques within schema therapy. In M. van Vreeswijk, J. Broersen, & M. Nadort (Eds.), *The Wiley-Blackwell handbook of schema therapy: Theory, research, and practice* (pp. 185–195). Chichester: Wiley.

3

Working to Connect Art Therapy on the Basis of Dialectical Behaviour Therapy for Clients Diagnosed with a Borderline Disorder

Outpatient treatment programmes for clients with personality disorders are increasingly adopting dialectical behaviour therapy (DBT) as a theoretical starting point. When working in a multidisciplinary team, this approach can be integrated into the various treatment components. For the art therapy component, this requires translation of the key aspects of DBT without impinging on the important theoretical principles underlying the art therapy itself. This translation has proved to be quite well possible in practice and provides a considerably better fit than initially expected.

3.1 What Is Dialectical Behaviour Therapy?

DBT is a broadly based cognitive behaviour therapy specifically developed for the treatment of people diagnosed with borderline personality disorders. The most important characteristic of dialectical behaviour theory is the assumption that the core disturbance in the borderline disorder is severe emotional dysregulation.

S. Haeyen, *Art Therapy and Emotion Regulation Problems*,
https://doi.org/10.1007/978-3-319-96773-8_3

The behavioural characteristics of individuals with borderline personality disorders can be regarded as effects of emotional dysregulation. Impulsive and, in particular, destructive behaviour can be construed as poorly adapted but nevertheless effective strategies for the regulation of emotions. Such strategies can, in the short run, reduce anxiety, provide distraction and mobilise help from the environment. Reliance on such maladapted strategies, however, clearly hampers the development of a stable sense of self and the normal expression of emotions. And such maladapted strategies for the regulation of emotions easily and frequently create confusion in relationships (Linehan, 1993, 1996).

Treatment for a borderline personality disorder is predominantly aimed at teaching clients to better regulate their emotions. In art therapy, four treatment modules can be distinguished parallel to the skills training components laid out in the DBT treatment programme.

- **Mindfulness**, one of the core ideas behind all elements of DBT. It is considered a foundation for the other skills taught in DBT, because it helps individuals accept and tolerate the powerful emotions they may feel when challenging their habits or exposing themselves to upsetting situations. The objective of mindfulness is learning to be in control of your own mind. (See mindfulness skills in the workbook.)
- **Distress tolerance** with the objective of learning to tolerate and survive crises and accept life as it now is.
- **Emotion regulation** with the objective of discovering, understanding and learning to deal with your emotions in a functional manner.
- **Interpersonal effectiveness** with the objective of learning to ask for what you need, learning to say 'no' and learning to handle conflict.

The four modules follow each other in a set cycle that allows the client to experience the themes addressed in the modules on two occasions within a treatment period of nine months. In the art therapy as I have given form to it within this treatment programme, each module is composed of a number of specific work methods which call upon the principles underlying DBT. The work methods can be found in the workbook in part two of this book. Use is further made of techniques from Gestalt art therapy (Rhyne, 1970, 1973a, 1973b, 2001) and Creative Problem Solving (Osborn, 2011).

Art therapy establishes a connection between the client's experience of the here and now and DBT. Via various mediums and methods for visual expression and representation, clients are helped to connect theory with their own experience. The therapist plays a coaching role here, leaving as much responsibility as possible to the client but at the same time offering structure as needed.

3.2 Dialectics

Just as the name suggests, DBT is based on a dialectical view of the world and reality. Reality is not viewed as static, but rather as consisting of internal opposing forces (thesis and antithesis). Out of the synthesis of these opposing forces, new opposing forces can emerge. This dichotomous and extreme thinking, behaviour and emotions so characteristic of borderline personality disorder is regarded as the result of dialectical failure or in other words, an incapacity to achieve some degree of synthesis. The individual is imprisoned in contradictions and is thus not able to move towards synthesis.

Two examples of the contradictions that may be experienced are:

- The necessity to accept yourself as you are but also the necessity to change at times.
- The stress and strain between getting what you want or need and losing what you want or need as a result of becoming more competent.

Dialectics entails the assumption that the fundamental nature of reality is change and development, rather than structure and content. As Linehan (1996) says: 'Change gives rise to both hope and anxiety. The objective of DBT is therefore to help clients feel more comfortable with the opposing forces in their lives. People seek to achieve greater balance, while the reality is that there will always be opposing forces at work. It is important to learn to live with opposing forces and to regulate them better' (Linehan, 1993, 1996).

3.3 Dialectics in Art Therapy

Dialectics is often visibly and concretely apparent in art therapy as what is expressed and creates tension and a dynamic. This is caused by opposing elements and is usually quite interesting to look at because of their interaction. Something can come across as open because something else is closed or, in other words, the presence of both elements is required for something to appear open or closed. Something looks big because some smaller elements are near it. Something looks complete because some loose or broken elements can be seen as well. Something is hidden but it can nevertheless be seen partly.

The dialectical principle fits nicely with the creative cycle of engagement, design, distance, reflection and then engagement again. A shattered figurine can elicit the initial reaction of judging it to be worthless and throwing it out. But stepping back and reflecting upon the broken pieces can lead to synthesis in the form of a new creative reaction with its own meaning. An initially aggressive, destructive impulse can thus make way for effective action: 'picking up the pieces' to make use of what has been broken.

Dialectics offers many starting points for art therapy to use specific work methods in working with polarities and contrasts. On the basis of contrasts in materials, methods and themes, a connection can be made to the inner conflicts being experienced by a client. By working through these conflicts and thus making contact with *both* sides of the underlying polarity, greater integration can be stimulated, and the objectives outlined later in this chapter can then be pursued. For example, a woman created drawings always showing her nice, soft and harmonious side in her contact with others. She typically works with pale, harmonious, flowing forms and pastel colours during art therapy. A focused exercise stimulated her to consider her 'dialectic' other side. The other side was drawn using bright, contrasting colours surrounded by thick, black borders. According to this client, this represented aggressive feelings. The goal of learning with dialectics in this example is to acknowledge and handle aggressive feelings and not trying to keep them out.

Art therapy interventions are aimed at the dialectic of accepting and confirming by giving concrete form but also eliciting change at the same time. This is achieved, for example, by asking the client to amplify a particular aspect of what has been created or to seek out its opposite.

Using the photographs presented here, I will illustrate how this dialectic manifested itself in the work of a number of clients (Figs. 3.1, 3.2, 3.3, 3.4, 3.5, 3.6, and 3.7).

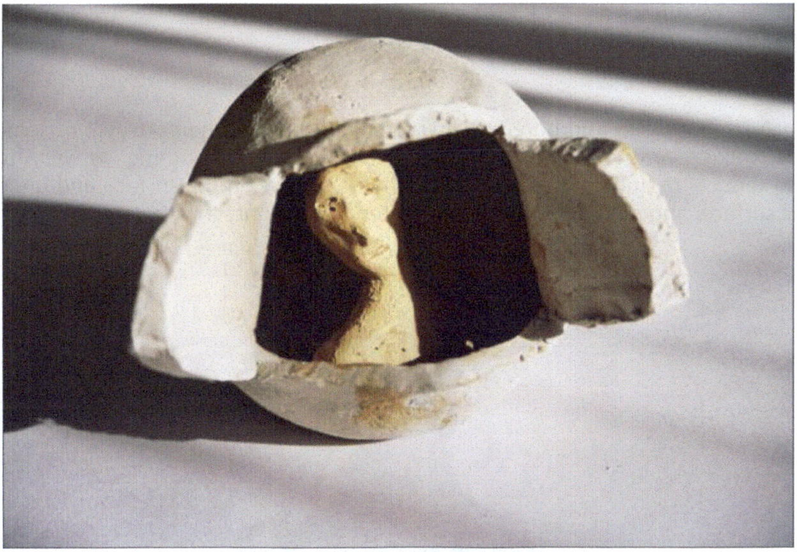

Fig. 3.1 This work communicates openness, but some reserve at the same time—depicted via the rounded form which can also be closed

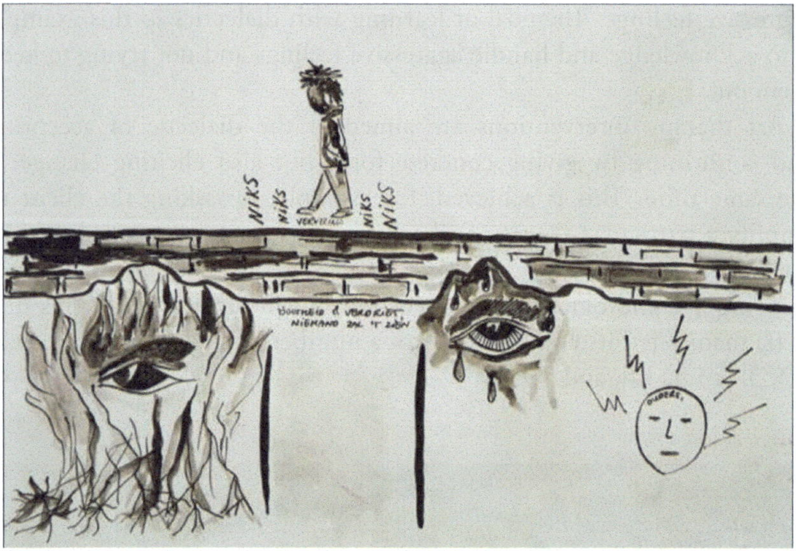

Fig. 3.2 Emptiness and boredom are communicated by the portrayal of someone walking on the surface in this work (see text: 'niks'/'nothing' as well) but also tension by the contrast between what is shown on the surface and under the surface: anger, sadness and stress related to the contact with parents

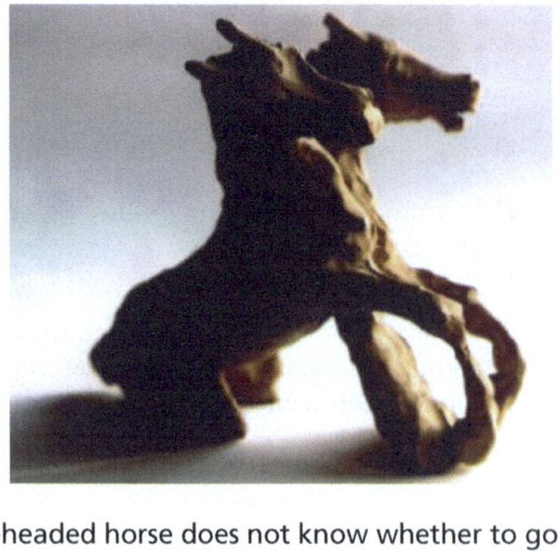

Fig. 3.3 The two-headed horse does not know whether to go left or right

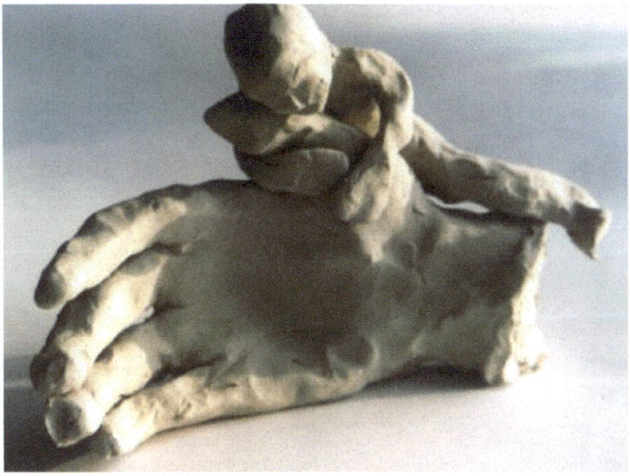

Fig. 3.4 The large hand represents responsibility and adult behaviour (acting independently) while, in contrast, the little figure appears to be searching for security and warmth

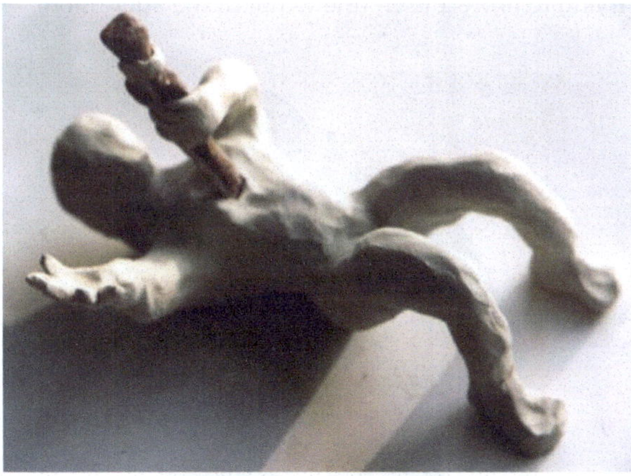

Fig. 3.5 The figure is sticking a dagger into its own heart but also, at the same time, reaching out a hand for help

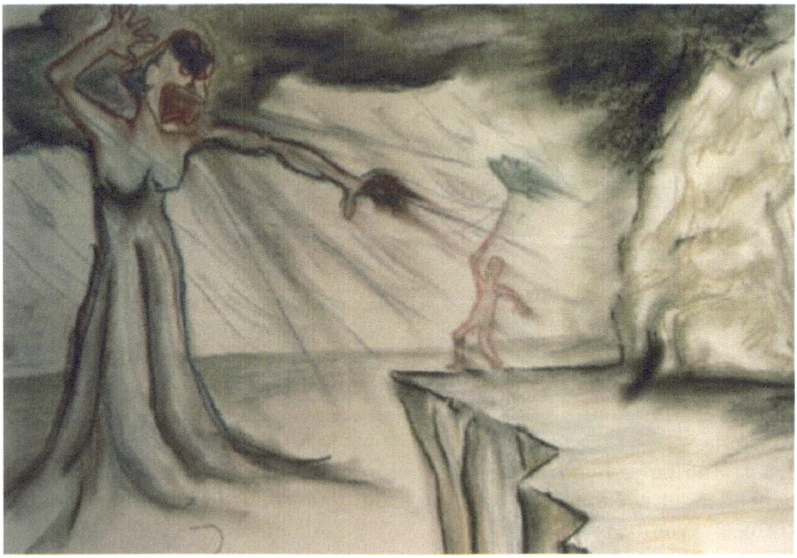

Fig. 3.6 The large figure (mother) is portrayed as a nasty aggressor across from a little figure trying to protect itself (the victim of the aggression)

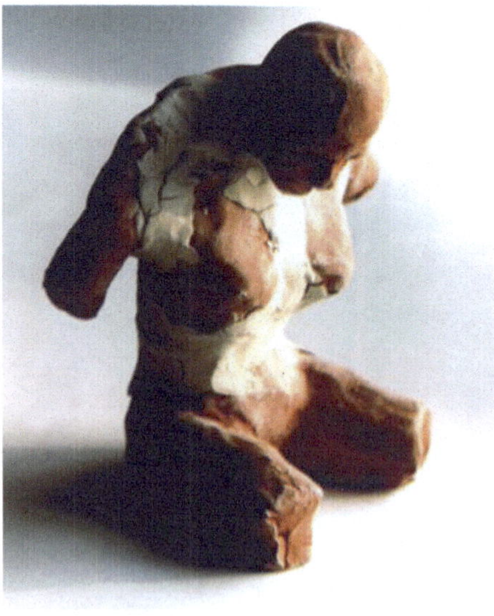

Fig. 3.7 The female torso which fell apart but was then healed/repaired. Both aspects can be seen

All of these examples illustrate dialectical dilemmas as they frequently occur in working with clients with borderline personality disorders. For the sake of completeness, I would like to emphasise that all of the interpretations and significance attached to the examples come from the follow-up discussions with the clients themselves and are thus what the clients actually said.

3.4 Objectives of Art Therapy Based on DBT

3.4.1 Learning to Express and Regulate Emotions

This takes place in the following manners.

- Expressing emotions in work produced during art therapy. This refers to emotional engagement in the work and participating with consciously focused attention (the here and now) and taking spontaneous action. At the same time, the emotion is structured by having the client translate it into a tangible, communicative work.
- Analyse what is being expressed in terms of:
  - Art process: describe how the work came about (self-observation), the creation of the work; during the process, keep attention focused and work effectively
  - Art product: what is there to see (observation)
  - Perception: observe and describe without being judgemental
  - Experience: describe your own feelings
  - Interpretation: non-judgemental, accepting
  - Redesign: either a new work is created or the existing work is altered on the basis of a revised vision, here too, focus attention and work effectively.

3.4.2 Achieving a More Stable Self-awareness

This takes place in the following manners.

- Accept your own art work and recognise its uniqueness.
- Expand your self-awareness by experiencing, discussing and analysing your own behaviour and work (for both individual and group works).
- Incorporate polarities from yourself into a single work; integrate polarities which stand for internal conflicts help achieve a sense of wholeness.

3.4.3 Practising with Interpersonal Skills

This takes place in the following manners.

- React to each other.
- Express the fact that you recognise something, identify with it.
- Give each other feedback.

Working together on assignments brings in interpersonal interaction (self-observation). Other social behaviour can be experimented with and practised as well.

3.4.4 Practising Distress Tolerance Skills

This takes place in the following manners.

- Call upon and challenge your problem-solving capacity by looking for additional and/or new artistic solutions.
- Gravitate to pleasant feelings in the work being created and then focus on this as a distraction from stress.
- Concentrate on acceptance.
- Concentrate on awareness and mindfulness.

This aspect involves experimenting with different materials, and openness and willingness to try out alternatives. The work method is comprised of an art problem, relaxation exercises and mindfulness exercises.

3.5 An Example: A Mindfulness Model

In what follows, I give an example of how DBT can be integrated into art therapy. This is done using a mindfulness model from the manual for DBT and training (Linehan, 1996). The skill training components for the other modules have been formulated in a similar manner (see the workbook).

The mindfulness skills provide a particularly good example of the skill training aspect of art therapy because mindfulness is central in DBT. The aim is to learn to be in control of your mind.

There are three mindfulness conditions or states of mind (see Figure, "Mindfulness model").

- The **rational or reasonable mind** is based on reason and logical thinking, on concentrating attention and calmly thinking about how to approach problems.
- The **emotional mind** steers thinking and behaviour primarily by the emotion of the moment. Thinking on the basis of reason and logic is difficult and everything is seen and felt emotionally.
- The **wise mind** integrates the rational and emotional minds but also goes beyond logical analysis and emotional experience to include intuitive knowing.

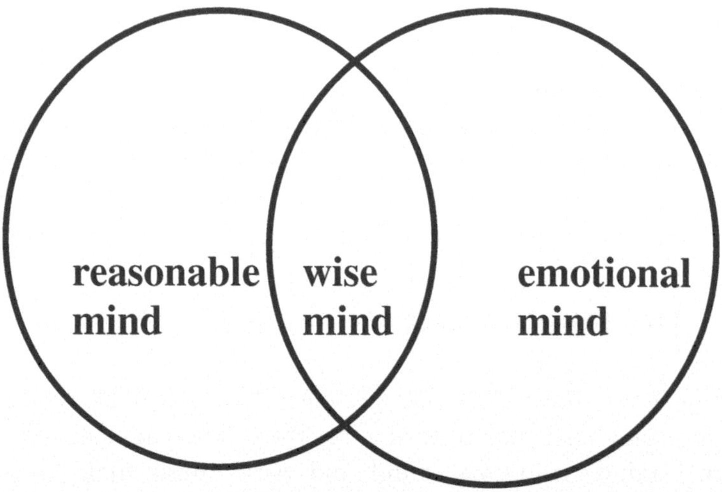

The Mindfulness model: three states of mind (Learning guide 1; Linehan, 1996).

The mindfulness skills help to bring the emotion and rational minds into balance and thus to reach the intuitive mind. The skills can be subdivided into *what* skills (observe, describe and participate) and *how* skills (non-judgementally, one-mindfully and effectively).

The What Skills

- Observing and paying attention to events, emotions and behavioural reactions without trying to stop them even when they are painful or trying to prolong them when they are pleasant. Learning to allow yourself to consciously experience a situation, no matter what happens, rather than trying to escape or put a stop to the emotion being experienced.
- Describing and labelling events and personal reactions and, as a result, gaining distance from emotions as opposed to becoming one with them.
- Participating and thus taking part without focusing on yourself. Acting spontaneously and attentively.

The How Skills

- Being non-judgemental or allowing perception without evaluation and thus nonbiased observation of behaviour and events.
- Doing one thing at a time; concentrating on that and not allowing yourself to be distracted by thoughts or images from the past, worries about the future or the presence of negative moods. Learning to control your attention.
- Acting effectively, aiming at what works, keeping objectives in mind and not acting against your own interests.

3.6 The Mindfulness Model in Art Therapy

At some point during art therapy, clients are asked to depict just how the three circles representing the three different states of mind (rational mind, emotional mind and wise mind) look for them personally. I ask them to visualise this using two equally large circles which overlap each other just as in the model. The material provided for this is pastel chalk, and the instruction is to work with line, form and colour. The main objective of an exercise such as this is to integrate the theory with the client's own experiential world. Remarkably, it often becomes apparent during this exercise just where a person's difficulties lie. In addition to becoming more aware of themselves, by creating and evaluating their work, clients gain practice with the specific what and how skills. In essence, clients are asked to participate spontaneously and with a clear focus during this assignment, to attend to one thing at a time, observe what happens, describe their own reactions, not to judge and to concentrate on what works (Figs. 3.8, 3.9, 3.10, and 3.11).

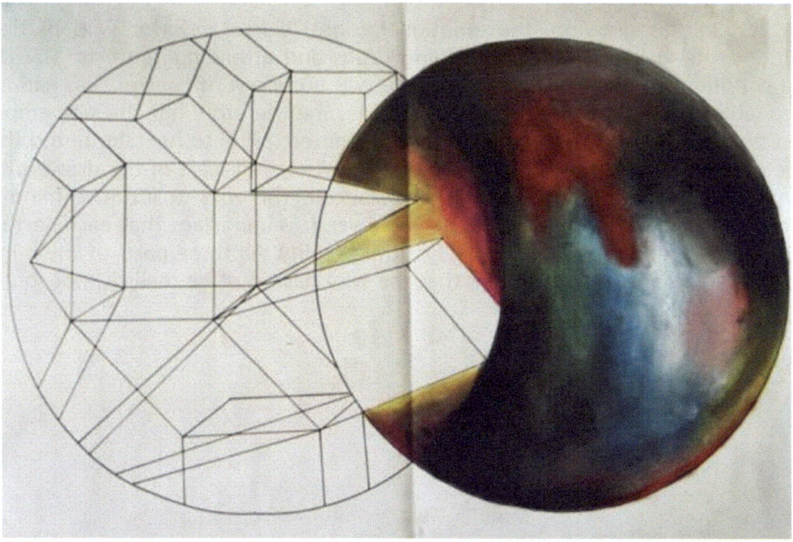

Fig. 3.8 Geometric constructions can be seen on the side representing the rational mind (left). The emotional mind depicts a rich but dark emotional world (right). The contrast between the two sides is quite marked. The two sides are brought together in the middle section representing the intuitive mind, but integration was apparently not possible

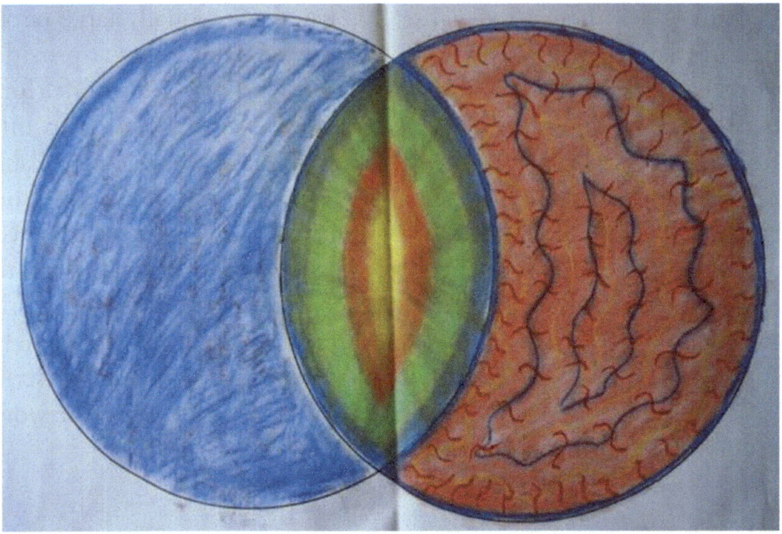

Fig. 3.9 In this drawing, the emotional (right) side stands for wild parties, fun and the kicks of going out, doing drugs and attending concerts. The client considered this 'real life', but her life was quite out of control. She had no idea what to draw for the rational (left) side. She therefore left this side empty and only coloured it solid blue, which represented 'calm' to her. She found this side of the drawing boring. She wanted the 'wise mind' part of the drawing to come across as beautiful, radiant and balanced. The wise or intuitive mind is often regarded as an ideal by clients. However, it is important that each part of the drawing represents some aspect of their reality. All three parts of the mind deserve acceptance, which means that the wise part must be realistic, not something unachievable

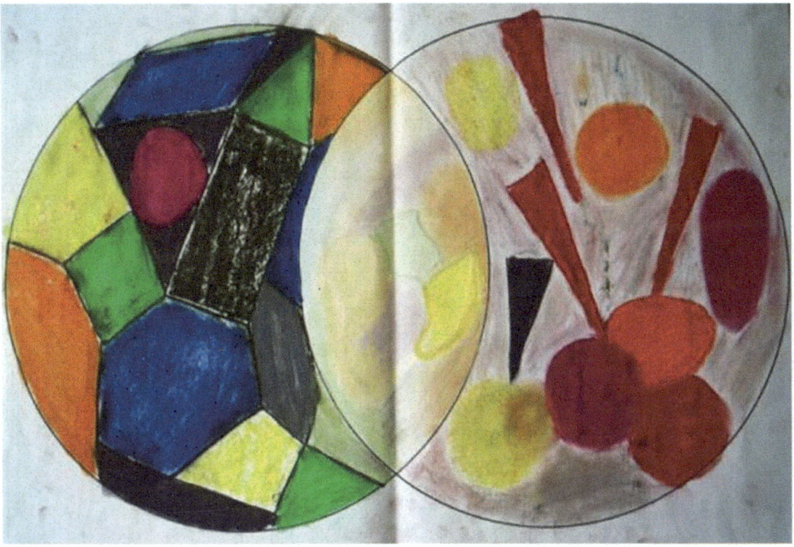

Fig. 3.10 This drawing was created by a man who comes across as very rational. Surprisingly, the rational side of the figure (left) is not as clean and straightforward as I expected on the basis of his behaviour. However, something is happening on the emotional side as well, where sharp, pointed forms are sticking into round forms. On this, the client said that it stands for feeling hurt, something that had happened frequently in the past and forcefully in the contact with this father. This hurt still determines the perceptions and behaviour of the client. He does not dare to show his feelings as he assumes that he will only get hurt again. The wise part of the figure is strikingly gentle, pale and light

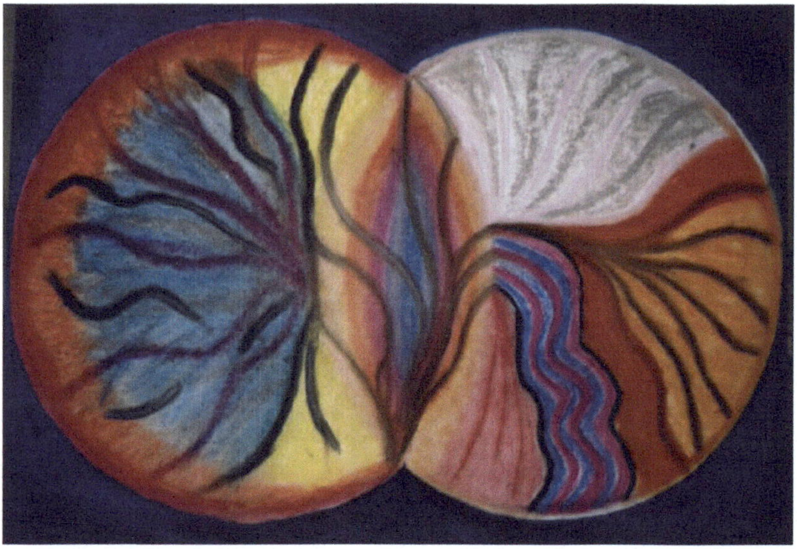

Fig. 3.11 This drawing was made by a woman who, at the start of therapy, showed mostly her rational side and liked to take on the role of co-therapist. In her own words, she could not 'get to her emotions'. Working on this exercise, she had to reflect explicitly on the emotional. While doing this, her face went from white to red and then she started to cry; she kept on working on the drawing until it was finished. She was so happy with the result depicting both sides of herself but the emotional side in particular, and the feeling of wholeness which this gave her, that she decided to take the drawing home and frame it for a place in her home. A very self-confirming experience!

3.7 Therapeutic Objectives

In art therapy incorporating key components of DBT, the following objectives are central: the client has gained greater insight into his or her emotions and learned to better regulate them. If these objectives are achieved, there will be less intense reactions to emotional issues, quicker recovery from intense emotions and reduced occurrence of unacceptable behaviour in response to experiencing strong emotions. The client manages to act in a manner which is more intentional and less emotion-driven. The client can better tolerate strong emotions and seek distraction when needed.

3.8 Conclusion

In addition to the value of DBT based on the content, it also has the major advantage of giving clients a therapeutic framework with clearly visible and recognisable treatment components. It integrates the therapy forms and promotes collaboration by the treatment team. The recurrence of familiar themes in different situations helps clients apply the theory to themselves with greater concentration. The experiences acquired during the sessions allow the theory to be applied directly and integrated deeply into the person. According to the clients themselves, 'When I hear or read the theory, I think: "likely, probably". But when I actually work with it during art therapy, I see clearly how it connects to myself; it is tangible, concrete'. This is the added value of art therapy in a treatment programme.

For myself, treatment is something dynamic and always in motion. I am constantly attuning the therapy to a given group of clients and the point at which they find themselves in their treatment.

As a team in the Expert Centre for Personality Disorders, we are always asking ourselves if what we are doing is good. This leads to the revision of existing modules but also to additions. These have come from the schema-focused therapy of Young (1994) as well as a specially developed skills training programme for emotion regulation. In short, reality is not static but rather, composed of opposing forces and polarities out of which synthesis can and should occur to give rise to new polarities.

3.9 Summary

This chapter has described an approach to art therapy which incorporates key components from the DBT of Linehan. The dialectic itself has been incorporated into the art therapy in different ways. It is inherent to the process of visualising what is being felt or thought and is evident in the methods adopted and the polarities they involve. Art therapy based on DBT is about learning to express and regulate emotions and achieving a more stable self-image, working on interpersonal skills and on distress tolerance. Seeing as experience is central in art therapy, they can better assimilate the theory underlying DBT than during other forms of therapy. Clients often say in this regard: 'When I hear or read the theory, I think: "plausible". But when I actually work with it during art therapy, I see clearly how it connects to myself; it is tangible, concrete'. This is the added value of art therapy in a treatment programme for borderline personality disorders.

References

Linehan, M. M. (1993). *Cognitive-behavioural treatment of borderline personality disorder*. New York, NY: Guildford Press.

Linehan, M. M. (1996). *Borderline persoonlijkheidsstoornisstoornis. Handleiding voor training en therapie* [Skills training manual for treating borderline personality disorder]. Lisse, The Netherlands: Swets & Zeitlinger.

Osborn, A. (2011). *Applied imagination: Principles and procedures of creative problem solving*. Milton Keynes: Lightning Source.

Rhyne, J. (1970). The gestalt art experience. In J. Fagan & L. L. Shepherd (Eds.), *Gestalt therapy now: Theory techniques applications*. New York: Harper & Row.

Rhyne, J. (1973a). The gestalt approach to experience, art, and art therapy. *Journal of the American Art Therapy Association, 12*(4), 237–248.

Rhyne, J. (1973b). *The gestalt art experience: Patterns that connect*. Chicago, IL: Magnolia Street Publishers.

Rhyne, J. (2001). The gestalt approach to experience, art, and art therapy. *American Journal of Art Therapy, 40*(1), 109–120.

Young, J. E. (1994). *Cognitive therapy for personality disorders: A schema-focused approach* (Rev. ed.). Sarasota, FL: Professional Resource Press.

4

Imagery in Art Therapy: A Schema-Focused Approach

It is a worthy objective, but not so simple to achieve: shaking off constraining patterns in the way you think, feel and act. As can be heard from Sly Stone (1969): 'Don't you know that you are free, well at least in your mind if you want to be'. Yet it is the objective of schema-focused cognitive therapy for personality disorders to change patterns in thinking, feeling and acting. This form of therapy works with experiential techniques, including guided imagery. In art therapy, internal imagery is followed by external imagery, or portrayal. What do clients think of this? Is it of help and how does it help them?

4.1 Introduction

In this chapter, I describe an imagery exercise in which clients work with their own experiences in the present and the past. It expands on an exercise based on the schema-focused therapy for clients personality disorders (Arntz & Bögels, 2000). I conducted this exercise with all my weekly therapy groups. In group art therapy, the images that arose, or

S. Haeyen, *Art Therapy and Emotion Regulation Problems*,
https://doi.org/10.1007/978-3-319-96773-8_4

certain aspects of them, were then worked out and portrayed using art materials. Afterwards, clients completed a questionnaire. Forty-eight of the 49 clients took part, and they all filled in the questionnaire. One client did not want to attend to this exercise.

I will first discuss a few basic terms used in schema-focused cognitive therapy for personality disorders and the role played by imagery. Then, I will describe the exercise and discuss the outcomes of the questionnaire I used to evaluate it. This is followed by the conclusions from the evaluation.

4.2 What Is Guided Imagery?

Imagery, or guided imagery, is a work form that starts with a relaxation exercise. After that, the therapist tells a story or sets down some guidelines on the basis of which participants can evoke their own images, atmosphere and fantasies.

Imagery can bring forward inner images that give expression to conscious or subconscious feelings, thoughts and desires. The imagery may focus on the past, the present, relationships with particular persons, future expectations or a person's self-image (Budde, 1989; McNiff, 2001). During an imagery exercise, participants are asked what they observe in themselves (through their senses, feelings and thoughts) and around them (colours, images, persons and surroundings) so that all aspects of an image and its effect on them as a person become clear. Imagery is one of several psychotherapeutic techniques that can open up deeper layers in the mind, that can delve beyond verbal and concrete behaviour. This is in part thanks to the fact that images belong to the inner domain, where people have the greatest degree of freedom and can be creative (Lusebrink, 1989; Taal, 1994).

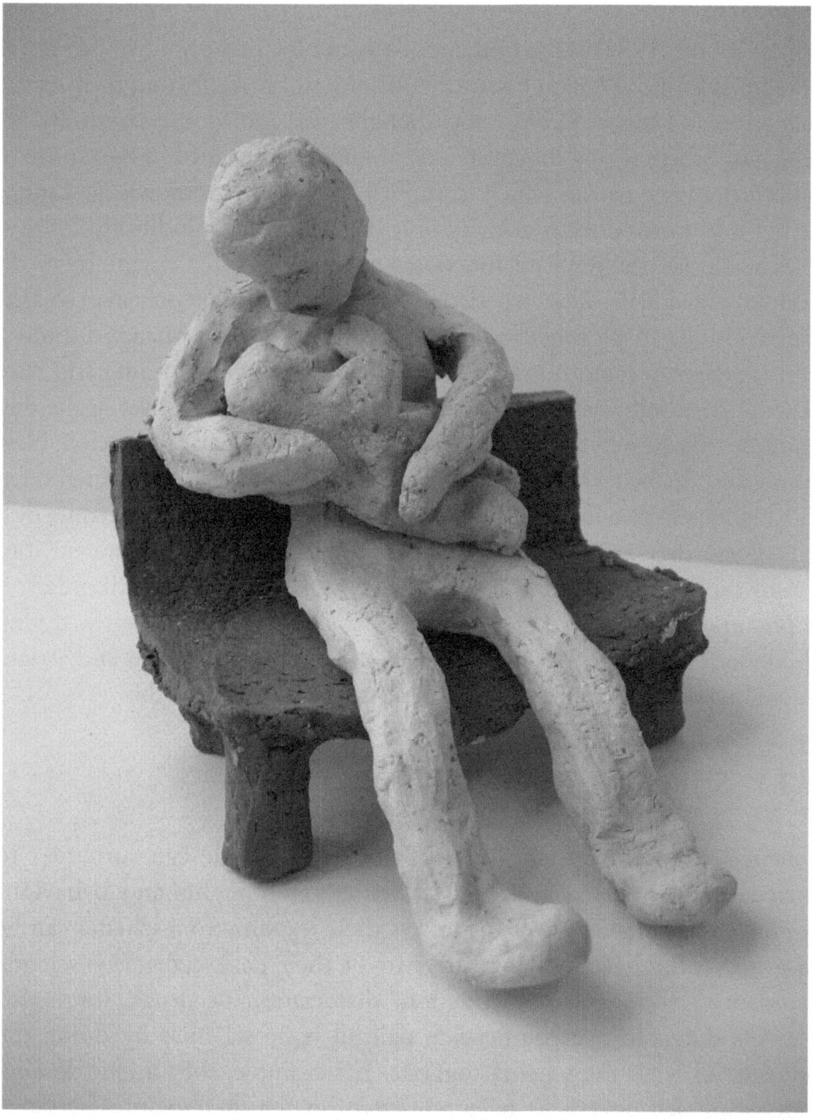

4.3 Schema-Focused Cognitive Therapy

Jeffrey Young (1994) is the founder of schema-focused cognitive therapy as developed for people with personality disorders. He starts from the premise that people's actions, feelings and thoughts are guided and controlled by schemas. Schemas contain collections of knowledge gained in the course of one's life, a large part of which is implicit. This implicit knowledge cannot be put into words directly and can only be reconstructed indirectly.

Schemas are the result of functional adaptation to the environment. In healthy individuals, new experiences can alter the older schemas so that they continue to be functional. In individuals with personality disorders, new experiences stand no chance: the schemas are so compelling and have become so firmly embedded by being repeated over and over again that new schemas, geared to new situations, have not been able to develop. New events and the behaviour of others are invariably perceived and interpreted in a highly selective manner. In other words, the schemas have become dysfunctional; they are no longer geared to the situation in the present, but simply replay situations from the past. In people with Axis II disorders, it is presumed that these dysfunctional schemas generally arise early, during childhood. Genetic disposition, interaction with central persons and certain intense events, such as traumatic experiences, may influence this.

4.3.1 Schemas in More Detail

Schemas can be active in a number of ways. People can surrender to their schema (schema surrender); then, their thoughts and behaviour confirm and enhance the schema. Or their response to a schema can be to avoid painful feelings that are part of their basic schemas—schema avoidance, by means of distraction, dissociation or drugs, for example. Or they can overcompensate painful basic schemas by doing the opposite of what the schema suggests. For example, they might develop narcissistic self-esteem as overcompensation for their painful sense of inferiority (schema overcompensation).

Schemas are not active all the time. A person may be able to function normally in a great many situations, and then suddenly panic and become clingy when faced with the possibility of being abandoned. Then, a schema is activated that takes over and controls the client's thoughts, feelings and actions. A schema that is so controlling is called a schema mode. Young describes eighteen basic schemas and four main types of schema modes (Young, 1994; Young, Klosko, & Weishaar, 2003). I will briefly discuss the schema modes below, linking them to borderline personality disorders:

1. The healthy adult mode
2. The child mode, in borderline clients often the angry child or the vulnerable child
3. The maladaptive protective mode, in borderline clients often the detached protector, disconnected from feelings
4. The internalised parent mode, in borderline clients often the punitive parent.

Cognitive therapy focuses primarily on building up more functional schemas and limiting the purview of dysfunctional schemas. If possible, the aim is at least partial personality change, in other cases smoothing or removing the sharp edges of the personality disorder pathology (Arntz & Bögels, 2000).

Therapy is formulated in schema mode terms, focusing on correcting the schemas from childhood and allowing them to develop, switching off the protective states (because they are dysfunctional) and replacing the internalised parent schemas (also dysfunctional because they are demanding, punitive or rejecting) by healthier schemas. Ultimately, the healthy adult schema will determine the greater part of a person's functioning. Giving schema modes a name and giving them a place (including a historic place) can provide guidance and support.

4.4 Imagery Exercise: Present–Past

4.4.1 The Nature of Imagery

Imagery is a technique used in cognitive therapy to clarify feelings and thoughts, to make links between recent events and experiences or perceptions from childhood, to lay bare dysfunctional basic schemas and to create newer, more functional schemas. Because imagery is primarily a non-verbal experience consisting of mental images, the newly created representations are felt more than thought. This is in keeping with personality disorders, which often have their origins in experiences from infancy and childhood, when the child had no one to confide in and was even not yet able to use language, for example, to take in or respond to his mother's reactions to him when he expressed his own emotions (Arntz, 2011, 2012; Arntz & Bogels, 2000).

Using imagery, schemas can be felt, recognised and named. This brings insight into the personal history of a person's schemas. At the same time, new experiences are created, and new experiences allow the schema to change. What takes place during an imagery exercise is advised to be put into words and given meaning, so that the new information is processed at all levels.

4.4.2 Target Groups

I carried out the imagery exercise called Present–Past (see the description later in this chapter and the complete description in the workbook entitled *Schema Therapy Module, Assignment 5*) in all my weekly therapy groups to investigate its usefulness and effectiveness. Afterwards, the clients completed a qualitative questionnaire. The following groups participated: three specialised groups for the treatment of personality disorders (primarily borderline personality disorders), an eating disorder group, two outpatient groups with mixed disorders (trauma, adjustment problems or mood disorders, neurotic disorders and less severe personality disorders), and an adolescent group (aged 17–23).

In the groups with personality disorders, schema-focused therapy is a module in the treatment programme, and the imagery exercise fits quite naturally in this module. In the other groups, the imagery exercise was integrated into the working method on a one-off basis.

4.4.3 Introduction to the Present–Past Exercise

Imagery techniques require good timing and supervision and need to be delivered by degrees, and it is important to place the exercise in a cognitive framework after completing it. The exercise is contraindicated if a person might decompensate. It is important to impress upon clients that they should not try to force images to appear, and that it is often wise to follow their first impulse, the first image that comes to mind. If clients repress an initial image, they often start to rationalise and lose touch with what they are doing.

During the exercise, it is important to let each person decide whether or not to close their eyes; fear of losing too much control must be kept manageable. The production of images may become blocked, and the point at which this happens is generally significant. During the exercise, intense emotions may come to the surface. It is important that emotions can be experienced; it is not a reason to stop earlier, unless a client wants to. The emotions can be given shape in the art work. This gives clients freedom to represent and put into words the experience and the feelings, so that they can be placed in a broader context. The result can be further examined during the discussion afterwards. This series of steps allows clients to feel the effects, and some processing may also take place.

4.4.4 Objectives of the Exercise

- Experiencing your own feelings
- Learning to describe experiences and express feelings
- Gaining insight by recognising links between feelings and thoughts that are part of the present and those that are from the past; recognising patterns and schemas
- Differentiating between present and past
- Working through and changing schemas, e.g. by calling up the healthy adult mode and making it active (step five in the exercise)
- Retaining/anchoring significant experiences and feelings as experienced during the exercise

- Opening yourself to the group in the form of personal art work and allowing others to participate in your experiences and feelings.

4.4.5 Instructions

Step 1. We start with a relaxation exercise focused on breathing and body awareness (duration around 5 minutes).

Then, the therapist says:

Step 2. 'Now try to imagine yourself in a pleasant situation in the present, one in which you feel very pleasant and safe. Where are you? Are other people with you? Who is there with you? What does this situation look like? What do you see around you? What do you feel? Is it hot or cold, are there particular smells? Let this situation sink in well. And once you have the situation well and clearly in mind, let go of it'.

Step 3. 'Now go in your thoughts to an unpleasant situation in the present. When did you feel unsafe, unsure? Are there others with you in this situation? Who is there? Where are you while this is taking place? What is happening, is anything said? What are your feelings? What do you feel physically? Are there any other things you notice in this situation? Once you have this situation clearly in mind, let go of it'.

Step 4. 'Now imagine yourself in an unpleasant situation when you were a small child. Wait and see if an image comes, don't force it. Look around you, at your surroundings, where you are and what it looks like, who is with you—is anyone with you?—and feel how it affects you. Look at the situation and at what is taking place, examine what you feel, and what you think'.

Step 5. 'Now imagine that you, the adult who you are now, that you walk into this situation. What would you do or say to help yourself as a small child, or to intervene? And then imagine that you actually do this. What happens, what is the response, or what changes in the situation? What do you feel? Make sure you have said and done everything you wanted to say or do. Is there nothing more you would like to say or do?'

Step 6. 'Now let go of this situation and go back to the pleasant situation in the present. Do you remember where you were? Try to see this situation clearly in your mind again. Feel what this situation does to you, what you feel'.

Step 7. 'Now gradually let go of this situation too. Bring your attention back to this room'.

(The imagery exercise takes around 10 minutes.)

Step 8. The creative assignment:

Portray a part, or several parts, of what you have imagined. Try to keep your attention focused on yourself. Choose whatever materials you like.

(The creative assignment takes around 45 minutes.)

Discussion

In the discussion, the focus is on people's experiences during the imagery exercise and the process of working creatively. We also look at the art works—at aspects such as form, content and perception.

The questionnaire is completed prior to the group discussion.

4.5 The Evaluation

Replies to the questionnaire

To clearly set down the positive and negative effects of the work form described above, and to help clients to order and retain their experiences, I gave all participants a questionnaire. This yielded a wide range of replies, as shown below.[1]

Question 1. Were you able to relax, and did the images arise spontaneously, or did they stop somewhere along the line?

The majority of the clients said they had been able to relax. The others had been unable to relax or only relaxed somewhat. A large majority of them (two-thirds) said that both the positive and the negative images arose spontaneously, and that these images often went straight to the heart of their problems. Sometimes, the images stopped briefly, and

[1]These are the answers as reported by the client, their own opinions and their own experiences. It should be pointed out that there were factors that influence reliability because the questionnaire could be completed in a socially desirable manner.

sometimes there were too many of them, so that they had to pick and choose.

Some clients did not want to allow negative images, primarily those from the past, because they were too painful. Sometimes, the process stopped at the positive experience in the present because their mood was too troubled. This seemed primarily to be the case in clients with mood issues such as depressive complaints.

Question 2. What memories came forward and what feelings and thoughts did they bring?

Positive experiences in the present were strikingly often situations near water (the sea, a boat and a holiday) and safe places such as in bed or on the sofa with pets. They also included contact with others (partner, friends and grandchildren) and one time, lying in bed in the parental home, a sense of briefly being a child again. They always revolved around experiencing peace and quiet, feeling safe and secure, relaxing, connectedness with no obligations, a sense of freedom.

Negative experiences in the present were situations in which they experienced a strong, onerous feeling such as sadness, shame, stress, loneliness or apathy. Such feelings were often caused by situations with others: an argument with the boss, a broken relationship, feeling punished/feeling shame or stress in contact with the other person. And sometimes it was the absence of a person that played an important role. One negative experience involved a recurrent dream of not-belonging.

The negative experiences in the past always went back to family situations and early school experiences. This often involved abuse, family arguments, being punished, sexually abused or bullied. Violent emotions were part of it: anger, loneliness, distress, impotence, feeling anxious, small and inferior. On the other hand, some participants had a strong focus on the emotions of the other: that person was not allowed to feel bad or be worried.

Question 3. What did you choose to portray and why?

The clients often chose to portray the unpleasant experience in the past, because it was the one that upset them most. Clients felt a great need to express their conflict-ridden perceptions, because that was where they saw the cause of their problems or where they encountered themselves. They wanted to see these perceptions on paper and view them from a distance. Sometimes, they chose to represent an experience from the past so as to avoid the most painful one (in this case the unpleasant experience in the present). When they chose to portray the pleasant experience in the present, people wanted to focus on the positive experience and the feeling it gave them, and to confirm and anchor this. Some chose to portray two or three situations because they were strongly interconnected.

Question 4. How did it feel, making this portrayal of your situation, and what strikes you in your work about how you portrayed it (What does it look like, what feeling does it express)?
Most clients said it gave them satisfaction to portray their mental images. Portraying the pleasant situation in the present always made them feel good. The feelings about portraying unpleasant situations were more diverse and often involved conflicting emotions. They often said they had a hard time making the representation because they were not sure how to portray all of the imagery or because they felt anger and sadness while they were working. One client said that she had found it difficult because it felt wrong somehow, like something that should not be exposed, but that she had still managed to make her portrayal show something.

Some clients felt that making the portrayal was less intense than the feeling the situation itself had given them; this came as a pleasant surprise. They enjoyed portraying their idea of what they would do as an adult in the situation from the past. Many clients were relieved to find that they could draw a clear boundary between past and present, thus separating and differentiating them. The groups produced a wide range of art works: some of them portrayed the actual situation, others made a symbolic representation, and sometimes their art work simply expressed their feelings in a more abstract manner using colour, line and movement.

Question 5. What is, for you, an important theme or an important feeling that came forward with the memories?
In reply, people often mentioned feelings of loneliness, anxiety, anger, powerlessness, sadness and feeling trapped. Several people said that showing and acknowledging emotions was an important theme.

Strikingly, in answering this question, a form of reflection took place in many clients, one that shows how they viewed their situation in retrospect. Some examples of answers:

> I now have what I wanted so badly in the past, a sense of security

> It's important that I try not to react the way I did in the past, even though I still tend to want to withdraw, to shut myself off

> Just let me muddle along in my own world, it's where I feel happy

This question also elicited doubts: 'Who am I?' and questions about the past: 'I wonder what my father was really like?'.

Question 6. When you entered the situation from the past as an adult, how did it make you feel, and what did you do?
Often, the adult offered consolation, responded to the child with understanding, hugged her and gave her hope. In a number of cases, the adult could protect the child against physical and/or mental violence by becoming angry, taking an assertive attitude or removing the child from the situation. This led to relaxation and relief. Sometimes, the adult's anger was so great that he 'could have killed' the other person. Clients who had been able to support or comfort themselves as a child, or to take positive action during the imagery exercise, said that it had been an important healing experience. One response: 'It was emotional, I walked over to myself as a child and put my arms around me, and just said, "go ahead and cry". This image moved me so strongly, the fact that I allowed myself to feel so deeply sad and forlorn'.

Comment: If we link this to the schema-focused therapy, we see that this client had the schema of a lonely, abandoned person, seen and comforted by no one. Now something had changed in her schema because she had experienced that she could console herself. One might say that the healthy adult was developing and learning to take care of the abandoned child in herself.

It would have been painful if the client, as an adult in the here and now, could only watch the unpleasant situation from the past and still be unable to do anything. In such a case, during the exercise, the client feels just as powerless and ensnared as in the past. The schema of the anxious, abandoned child is then active, and it is not possible to call up a healthy adult mode.

A few times the adult acted in a way the client was not really satisfied with. This was the case, for example, when the adult picked up the child and fled, or made sure that no one could find anything to criticise in her (a protective mode aimed at adaptation).

Question 7. What did this exercise give you?
Many clients felt it was a very meaningful exercise because it gave them insight and they could come to terms with certain feelings:

> I always felt alone, and in fact I still do. If only there was someone who put an arm around me and said that everything would be all right.

> In unpleasant situations in the present, the pain from the past comes back, I'm still alert and anxious, I feel a lot of anger – what belongs to the past and what belongs to the here and now?

> In the past, my parents were just not there for me; I felt abandoned by them. Now, when they ask me to do something for them, I'm extremely abrupt; now I am not there for them either.

A few clients discovered that they now in fact have something they had lacked in the past and always wanted to have. This awareness gave them a sense of appreciation of what they now have, as can be seen in Figs. 4.1 and 4.2.

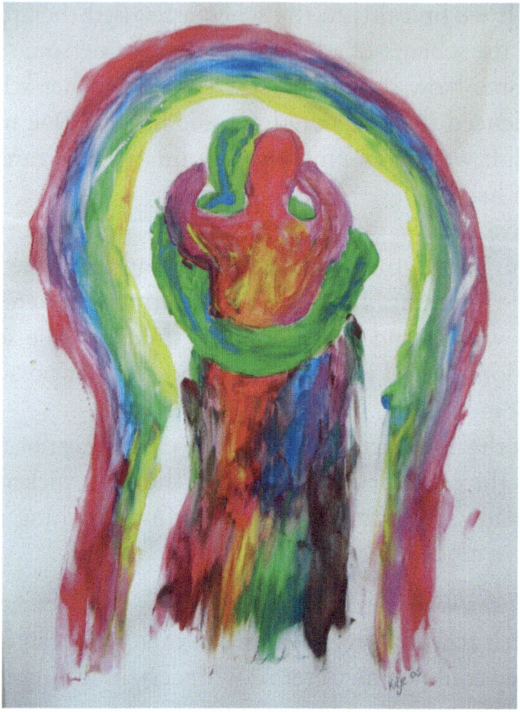

Fig. 4.1 I finally realise that now I feel the warmth in my relationship that I so sorely missed in the past

Other clients pointed out being confronted by 'thinking about things that you don't normally want to think about' or that make you realise that 'you haven't come as far as you thought in your treatment'. This feeling served to strengthen the will to change.

The clients gained more insight into differentiating between then and now, or they recognised similar patterns in the past and the present.

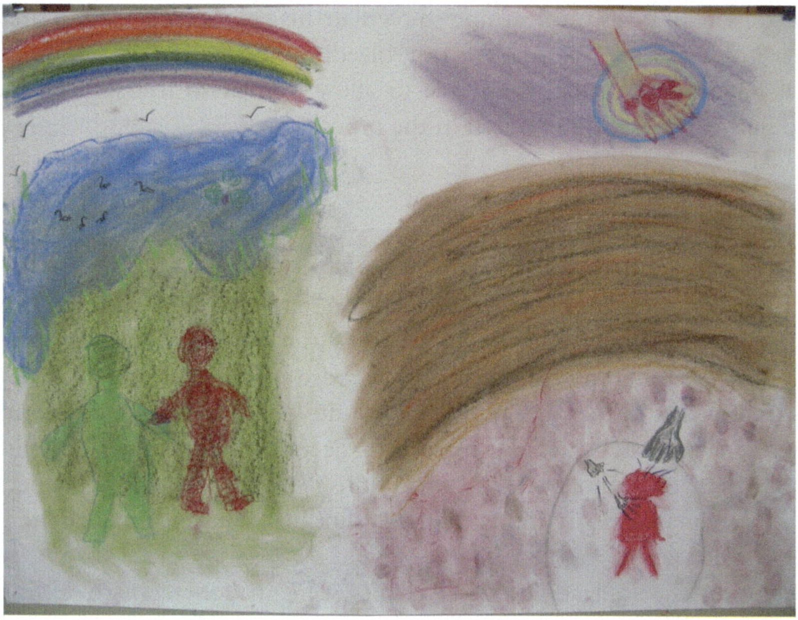

Fig. 4.2 Differentiating between, and seeing the relationship between, past and present; on the right, being smacked as a child, but also in the top right-hand corner, the guardian hand of herself as an adult. At the left, we see her situation now: harmoniously strolling with her partner. Her basic schema is that she often feels deserted and inferior

Clients could choose which aspects they wanted to spend more time on—for example, a positive experience or an aspect laden with conflict. This choice can be examined later, and it provides opportunities for interventions.

Sometimes, someone does not want to take part, for example, Keith, 39 years old. He said: 'If I do, I will become very aggressive and I'm afraid I won't have myself under control'. He wanted to be an onlooker. So he stayed and watched, but even so, images came to mind. Despite being frightened and anxious at the sadness and anger he felt at seeing these images, he decided to portray them in an art work because one of his treatment goals was learning to regulate his emotions. Out of a small piece of soapstone, he made a tiny bleeding heart. He was emotional, but happy that he had been able to allow himself to feel some of his feelings without losing himself in the process.

4.6 Conclusion

The evaluation shows that the imagery exercise and its subsequent portrayal are useful and effective in attaining the objectives, such as experiencing and identifying schemas that arose in the past and that now restrict clients in the present. Clients could feel, recognise and describe their basic schemas and the place they occupied in their personal history. They also came to see connections between earlier experiences, basic schemas and situations that they find difficult and unpleasant in the present.

During the imagery exercise, clients were in contact with feelings related to the child mode. The healthy adult mode was evoked to intervene in a situation, and this could bring about a change in the schema. This process was reinforced by portraying it in an art work. Clients found this exercise meaningful. The images that came to mind yielded a great deal of material for the treatment process and for therapeutic interventions. By portraying this in art therapy, they gained a new opportunity—being able to make their own choices, to distance themselves—and they were encouraged to again reflect on their experiences and their art works. This represents being able to separate and differentiate present and past but also to see relationships between present and past. Significant experiences were fully felt, confirmed and anchored, both by retaining positive feelings and by meaningful experiences such as being able to intervene as an adult in an experience from the past. It clarified many things that had been less clear before, it made palpable and visible what schemas were involved and how the change in a schema looks when portrayed on paper, and thus what form this change can take in a client's daily life.

4.7 Summary

Schema-focused therapy for personality disorders, developed by Jeffrey Young, works with experiential techniques, including imagery. It provides a framework for art therapy to work with concrete, personal experiences and to investigate the underlying schemas. After the imagery exercise, the next step is expressed internal images in an external form using art materials. This makes it possible to anchor, confirm and reflect on these images. This chapter is a summary of the main findings from clients who carried out an imagery exercise and then portrayed their findings in an art work. Their findings show that the objectives were attained and that the creative aspect added essential elements.

References

Arntz, A. (2011). Imagery rescripting for personality disorders. *Cognitive and Behavioural Practice, 18,* 466–481. https://doi.org/10.1016/j.cbpra.2011.04.006.

Arntz, A. (2012). Imagery rescripting as a therapeutic technique: Review of clinical trials, basic studies, and research agenda. *Journal of Experimental Psychopathology, 3,* 189–208. https://doi.org/10.5127/jep.024211.

Arntz, A., & Bögels, S. (2000). *Schemagerichte cognitieve therapie voor persoonlijkheidsstoornissen.* Houten and Diegem: Bohn Stafleu Van Loghum.

Budde, E. (1989). *Creatieve therapie in praktijk.* Deventer: Van Loghum Slaterus.

Lusebrink, V. (1989). Art therapy and imagery in verbal therapy: A comparison of therapeutic characteristics. *American Journal of Art Therapy, 28,* 2–3.

McNiff, S. (2001). The use of imagination and all of the arts. In J. A. Rubin (Ed.), *Approaches to art therapy: Theory and technique* (pp. 318–325). New York: Brunner-Routledge.

Stone, S. (1969). *Stand!* [Album]. Redwood City: Epic.

Taal, J. (1994). Imaginatietherapie. *Tijdschrift voor Psychotherapie, 20*(4), 227–246.

Young, J. E. (1994). *Cognitive therapy for personality disorders: A schema-focussed approach* (Rev. ed.). Sarasota, FL: Professional Resource Press.

Young, J. E., Klosko, J., & Weishaar, M. (2003). *Schema therapy: A practitioner's guide.* New York: Guilford Press.

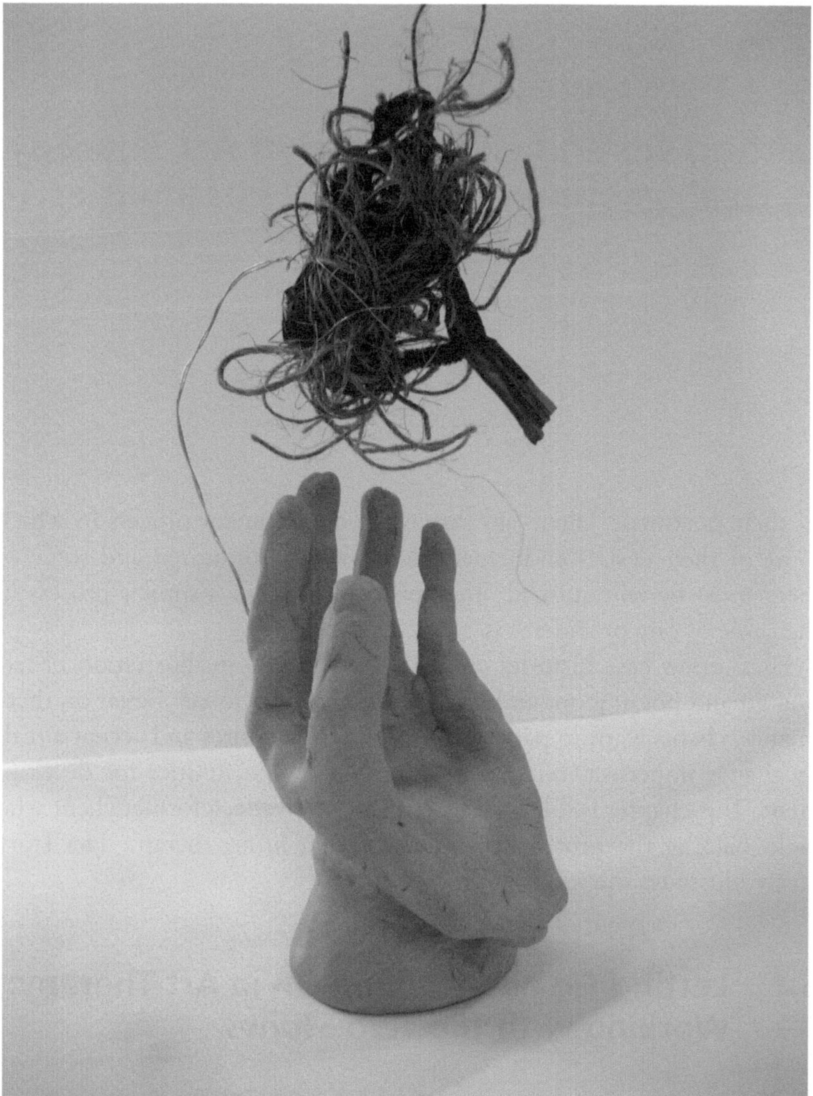

5

Letting Go and Holding On in Art Therapy: Disillusionment and New Possibilities

In their treatment, clients go through a development process in which some of their desires and expectations can be confirmed and some of them must be relinquished. Therapists go through a similar process in their role of care provider.

First, a few case histories are briefly recounted in illustration of letting go and holding on, and interventions are discussed. Based on these themes, clients learn to part with some of their desires and accept a reality that is imperfect, but which offers new opportunities for development. This chapter is followed by the story of Katie, a former client who looks back at the process she went through in art therapy. Her story nicely illustrates the subject of this chapter.

5.1 Letting Go and Holding On in Art Therapy: Working with *the Two Stones*

Numerous letting go processes are inevitably part of art therapy. Multatuli described 'An illusion lost is a truth found' (Stuiveling & Van den Bergh, 1995) which is a dialectic and also hopeful perspective.

S. Haeyen, *Art Therapy and Emotion Regulation Problems*,
https://doi.org/10.1007/978-3-319-96773-8_5

If a person wants to change something, it is very likely that something will have to be let go to achieve that change. Every change has its price. The behaviour to be changed served a certain purpose. It may have filled a void or yielded attention. This asks for a new point of view, a new orientation. Do I really want to change? What will I have to give up? Do I really want to do that? In investigating and focusing on choices—what a client wants to hold on to and what to let go of or change—one of the work methods I use is *The two stones: holding on and letting go* (see the workbook module *Emotion regulation, assignment 17: Two stones—holding on and letting go*).

After an exercise in imagination, clients paint two stones; one stone shows what the client wants to leave behind and the other what he or she wants to keep. They are also given homework: they take both stones home with them along with a special assignment. The assignment is, within the next few days, to consciously and deliberately throw away the first stone (which represents letting go) or leave it behind somewhere. For the second stone (which represents holding on), they must find a place to keep it where they can see or feel it. This encourages the transfer of their experience in art therapy to their own daily routine. By literally throwing away the first stone they painted, which has become a symbol of some aspect of their life, certain feelings come to the surface; clients are confronted with the emotion that accompanies letting go.

Some Case Histories

A few weeks ago, client Alma attempted suicide after an argument with her boyfriend. She is often involved in aggressive incidents, and her language can be blunt and coarse. She pays little attention to her emotional—vulnerable—side and has little contact with it. She says she finds it important to develop this, and so it is one of the main goals of treatment for her. But then, she will need to let go of her rough outer veneer, her tough presentation of herself. During art therapy, she shows some guarded growth, but a feisty, uninterested attitude is still manifest. On the stone showing what she wants to let go of, she paints a middle finger. It stands for anger, for toughness and for conflicts with certain people in her life. On the other stone, she paints what she wants to keep: a red heart. She explains that she wants to hold on to the fact that she now realises (after her suicide attempt) that there are more people around her who love her more than she thought. She had thought that no one really cared.

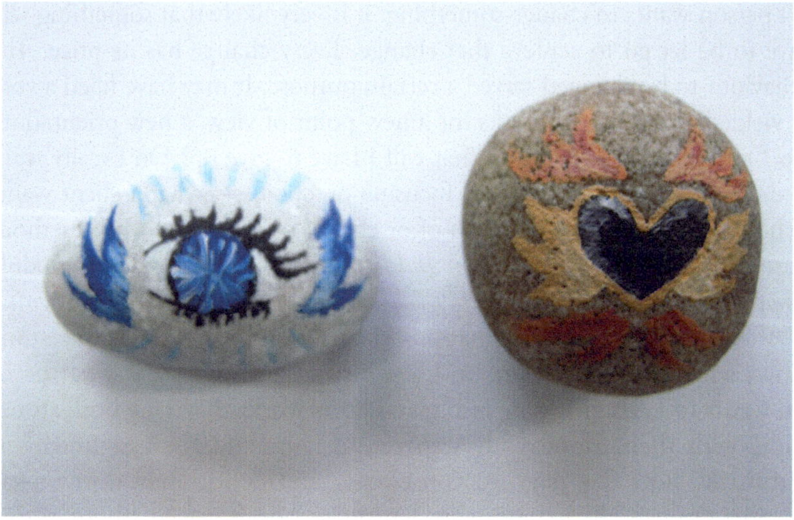

Fig. 5.1 The two stones of Ilona

In the past, client Ilona had a number of unpleasant relationships in which she was abused and allowed herself to be used sexually. She has a symbiotic relationship with her mother. On the stone she wants to let go of, Ilona makes an image of a black heart with wings. It symbolises the poor relationships she has had, relationships that have damaged her. She no longer wants such relationships. She wants to hold on to what she has learned: to let her emotions, her intuition and speak more. She portrays this in a shining pale blue eye (Fig. 5.1).

A week later, she says that she has not yet got rid of the first stone. Straightaway, her mother said, 'But it's so lovely! Surely you won't throw it away?' This made it quite difficult for her, but she realises that she does want to get rid of the stone, despite her mother's reaction. This has given the stone even greater significance: Do I make my own choices or do what my mother wants?

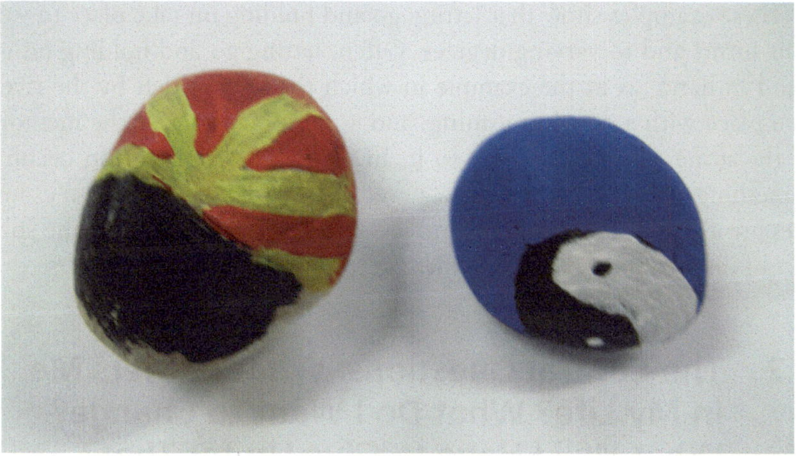

Fig. 5.2 The two stones of Sarah

Client Sarah leads a wildlife and regularly freaks out just for kicks. Aggressive incidents are a familiar occurrence. In her treatment, she wants to learn to let go of her impulsiveness, but then again, she gets a great kick from that side of her (Fig. 5.2).

While I explain that, after painting the stones, the homework will be to deliberately get rid of the first stone, she immediately becomes extremely anxious. She says so, and we can see it: her face has gone completely red. At the same time, it takes her by surprise. My comment that choosing to let go of her impulsiveness was perhaps a rational decision, but not at an emotional one, hits home. She agrees that this may well be the case. She thinks it might be better to wait a while before letting go of the stone, until she can stand behind this decision, and for now, just to put the stone someplace where she can always get it back again.

Another client, Muriel, knows when she starts painting exactly where she will leave this stone. It is a place by the river she often went to as a child. She wants to put the stone in the water there. A week later, she has. She even took a picture of it and is very content. The other stone is at home in a nice safe spot.

These examples show that letting go and holding on take place in various forms and to varying degrees. Often, letting go and holding on go hand in hand, as in the example in which the stone is left by the river, in a place with a certain meaning, and a photograph keeps the memory of the stone alive, holding on to it. In this way, letting go can become something that is held and kept, never to be forgotten. All these examples are about choices, about central issues that are continually the subject of discussion in the treatment.

5.2 The Central Questions: What Bothers Me in My Life? What Do I Want to Change? What Will I Have to Give Up for That? and Is That What I Really Want?

Going into therapy means that something bothers you, and that you want to change it, or that you feel it is necessary. Whether the change you have in mind is realistic and attainable is also important. During the therapy, the wish to change becomes more concrete, and the price to be paid for it becomes clearer. Old behaviour must be abandoned, certain thoughts or feelings lose their validity. And still, there was a reason for this behaviour, these thoughts or feelings. They had, and still have, a function: they provide you with something.

Feelings of loneliness and disconnectedness, for example, are reasons to go into therapy, if a person wants to change and perhaps have more contact with others. A client may placate her unpleasant feelings by telling herself that she is very special—and that is why she has so few friends. Here too, being in therapy means letting go of your own personal flattery and investigating where you can feel acknowledged by and connected with others. A life full of kicks may counter some feelings of emptiness and sombreness. It gives you a facade of being an exciting and 'cool' person. Going into treatment may then mean accepting that your life will be calmer, even 'boring'.

Being in therapy fundamentally means that a process is taking place in which a person's self-image is changing; it means, for example, letting go of the ego-ideal or the false self-image and developing a realistic self-image; moving from huge demands to attainable goals, from escapist behaviour (drugs and kicks) to starting to feel, to allowing yourself to feel; from letting down your facade and accepting your own vulnerability; from holding on to the victim role to taking responsibility, perhaps even facing up to your role as a culprit; taking leave of idealised images of parents, wishes and desires that are still problematic; and turning them into more realistic pictures of parents in which they have their limitations like everyone else.

Not infrequently, this process requires a non-traumatic disillusionment. What this means: the idealised self-image or image of the other is dismantled in a way that it is not harmful; it is not an upsetting confrontation, but one that takes place gradually, in which there are understanding and respect for the client's perception, so that the client can find a new way of connecting to reality that is acceptable to him or her.

5.3 The Process of Letting Go and Holding On, of Change and Acceptance

So that clients are aware of, and thinking about, the central questions (What is bothering me? What do I want to change and what will I have to give up for that? Is that what I really want?), and to foster the process of letting go and holding on, it is important to let them investigate what they want to change, what would be a realistic self-image, and what may stand in the way of change. It is important that clients make their own choices that they are encouraged to do so and take responsibility for it. The therapist is not making a moral judgement, not even a suggestion, but explaining what options there are and placing responsibility with the client.

In this regard, it is enabling for clients to become keen observers, to analyse situations with a focus on their own thoughts, conduct and feelings. People diagnosed with personality disorders often have trouble with this. They easily fall prey to cognitive deformations, to impulsive and emotional interpretations.

The therapist works towards both acceptance and change, according to the dialectical principle that reality consists of contrasting forces in an ongoing dialogue. This theme fits in withholding on (acceptance) and letting go (change). The therapy focuses on examining and expressing unfulfilled desires or feelings, and concluding or finalising them. Clients learn to regulate feelings by allowing them and then letting them go, by being in charge of their figurative emotional faucet.

The therapist, too, must face up to her own illusions and focus on identifying them. Some clients choose to hold on to illusions. They continue to let their actions be guided by their emotional mind and are unable to integrate the emotional thinking mind and the rational thinking mind into the wise mind. This may have far-reaching consequences, and sometimes only comes forward at the end of treatment, which is a confrontation with reality for the therapist. Some clients continue to function in a more isolated or limited manner than the therapist had expected or hoped for. Lastly, letting go of the client at the end of the therapy is not always easy. The therapist has committed him/herself to the client and now must say goodbye to him or her.

Attention to the end of the therapy is thus important for both parties, both for clients and for the therapist. Consciously saying goodbye, taking time for this, relying on a ritual, these can all be ways of recognising and acknowledging this process of letting go of the therapy, of the group and of fellow members, of each other as client and therapist.

5.4 Holding On to Experiences from Art Therapy

One of the starting points of therapy is that what clients experience in therapy influences and changes their lives outside therapy, that their experiences are transferred from one situation to the other. As the therapist, you might assume that experiences are transferred automatically. After all, art therapists assume there is an analogy between what takes place in the medium and behaviour, between thinking and feeling in everyday situations. But the question is still whether this actually takes place, at least to a sufficient extent. Transfer can be encouraged, and it is probably too important not to deliberately push for it. This is a good reason to pay special attention to the process of holding on to the experiences gained in art therapy.

5.4.1 Transfer and Art Therapy

Some examples of ways to encourage transfer in art therapy:

- Making concrete links between producing works and day-to-day reality by portraying 'real' or realistic situations and the client's present feelings in assignments.
- In the discussion afterwards, actively making verbal links to daily practice (patterns of behaviour, thinking and feeling on analogy with working in the medium), asking 'Do you recognise what is happening here in other situations as well?' and 'What could this experience offer you in other situations?'. This also makes the transfer from the experience gained to articulating it (cognitive processing/framing/placing in a broader context).
- Giving assignments focusing on transfer as their objective:
  - Homework assignments (address themes in your own practice situations, involve surroundings and give written assignments for in between therapy sessions).
  - Make a symbol or an expressive flashcard to focus on a thought or an object (e.g. see the workbook module *Distress tolerance skills, assignment 5: Helpful symbol.*
  - Have clients, take their work home to display somewhere, throw away or keep as a memento, perhaps by taking a photograph of a work to take home (a cell phone photograph or an instant picture such as a Polaroid snapshot).
  - Use photographs from your own album/records or self-written texts on which to base a work. A work based on photographs takes on a new personal meaning in the light of the therapeutic objective (e.g. see the workbook module *Schema-focused therapy*, assignment 7: Picture then and now).
  - Rituals to give personal shape to letting go and holding on.
- Working with the client's family or partner so that they can practice behavioural change in the home surroundings, or so that feelings can be processed there.

But sometimes you don't want the therapeutic situation to be too much like the concrete, day-to-day private situation; you want to offer greater scope, more freedom so that clients can experiment with different behaviour. Because they are creating art works, this is already a different perspective; they are often not accustomed to produce work like this at home or to look at problems from such a perspective, let alone work on them. The art medium offers a form of protection which allows difficult feelings to be there. What is veiled in the medium while working can be articulated and placed in a broader context during the discussion afterwards, and transfer to the private situation can be stimulated.

The figure shows how the client's own private situation and art therapy come together in the overlapping circles:

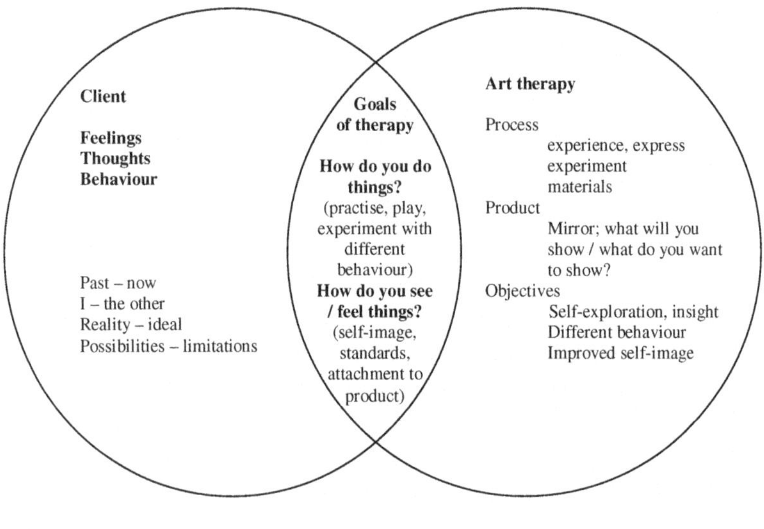

5.4.2 Rituals

Art therapy offers many possible ways of dealing with themes related to holding on and letting go. One way is the use of a ritual. Rituals sometimes have a fixed form (e.g. a leave-taking or farewell ritual, see the workbook module, *Special situations, assignment 9: What do you take with you..(…) and 10: Goodbyes*). A fixed form or pattern gives guidance and grip and has a unifying effect in a group. Sometimes, for example, when clients want to work on a more personal theme, it is important that they can choose the form themselves. A transitional ritual is a means of reinforcing a passage from one period to the next. The experience is transferred, and a ritual makes this concrete and visible. Rituals signify special moments and are often characterised by activities (doing something special, something suitable and symbolic, such as burning, burying, giving away or framing), saying something, giving a speech (your own text, a poem and something with distinct significance), there is a focus on objects (works and personal items) and sometimes there are witnesses (therapist, group members, friends or family). Often, some reminder is kept to commemorate it (an object such as a souvenir, a photograph and a work).

Case: 'Treasure Chest Framed in Gold'

Client June wants to do something with the painful feelings surrounding her life, her adoption, her problems with her adoptive parents, her negative self-image and the fact that she does not allow herself to have a successful life. It is a wide-ranging and comprehensive goal, but bit by bit, these matters come up in the therapy. At a certain point, she brings some photographs the group had asked to see. They are pictures of her as a baby, tiny and crying. She makes a collage of the photographs. Over it, she places a picture of a treasure chest (see Fig. 5.3). The treasure chest covers the collage; the collage is not always visible, but people can see it by peeping inside the treasure chest. This symbolises how she wants to deal with the matter: it's there, but I don't want it to be too obvious, I don't want it to play such a big role. She has found a lovely saying to go with it: 'I don't know if I can love the desert, but it is the desert that hides my treasure…'. She puts the treasure chest in a gold frame she has brought with her and takes the work home, where she puts it in a prominent place. In this way, she gives shape to a troublesome and wide-ranging theme and gives it a place in her life.

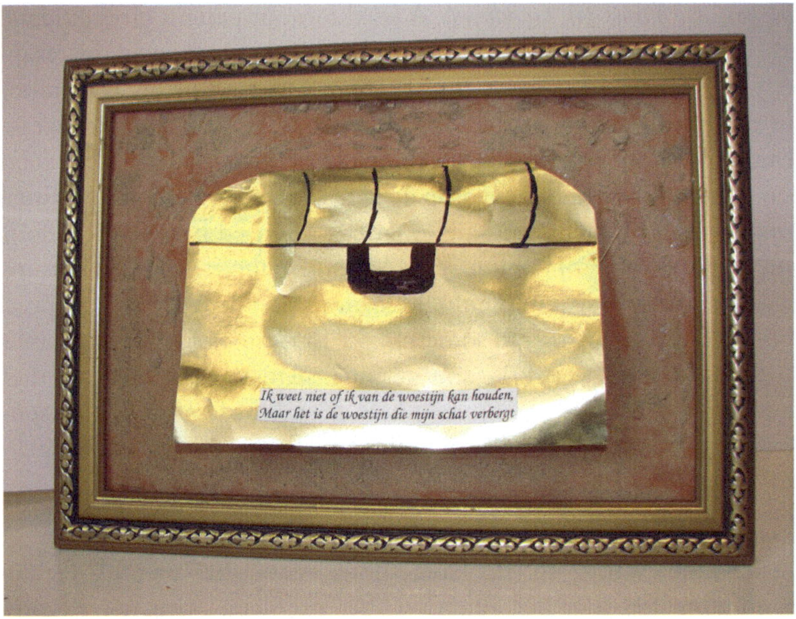
Ik weet niet of ik van de woestijn kan houden,
Maar het is de woestijn die mijn schat verbergt

Fig. 5.3 The treasure chest

5.5 Integration: Transfer Between Parts of the Self

Bringing together, linking and integrating different parts of the self that are miles apart can be an important objective in art therapy. This can involve working out different polarities in the person, but also unravelling various positions or schemas that are active. The latter fits in well with Young's schema-focused therapy (1994; Young, Klosko, & Weishaar, 2003) and with Transactional Analysis (Berne, 1961). It is also found in Gestalt therapy (Rhyne, 1970, 1973a, 1973b, 2001): by making contact with both sides of the polarity (in yourself), particularly with the side with which you do not usually identify, an opportunity arises for integration, bringing yourself together. The story of former client Katie that follows this chapter is a good and meaningful example. In her process, her various sides start to communicate with each other, and this brings her to integration.

5.6 Encouraging Transfer in a Broader Context

In addition to the art therapy, gearing the various aspects of multidisciplinary treatment as closely as possible also encourages transfer by using a consistent and shared framework. According to outcomes of research by Bateman and Fonagy, this is an important factor in the effectiveness of integrated therapies. Their conclusion is that no one method is superior in this context (Bateman & Fonagy, 2006; Landelijke Stuurgroep Multidisciplinaire Richtlijn ontwikkeling in de GGZ [National Advisory Committee Regarding Multidisciplinary Guidelines for Development in Mental Healthcare], 2008).

It also promotes transfer within the treatment if the various treatment aspects refer to one another where appropriate. A particular theme can perhaps be covered very well by letting the client work on it in another aspect of therapy too. This builds bridges, makes connections between the therapy aspects and the various experiential areas.

Transfer to the client's immediate environment may be encouraged by family discussion groups or family treatment and by holding general information meetings about the treatment with some regularity for family and/or friends of the client, so that the client's surroundings become involved in his or her change process.

5.7 Summary

Letting go and holding on in art therapy is an important theme that comes up in all manner of forms and at all levels. At an intrapsychic level, it revolves around the central questions in the therapy: What is the problem? What do I want to change? What will I have to forego? Is that what I really want? These questions are related to the theme of transfer: what do I want to take with me and what will I let go of or leave behind. It is important to consciously encourage transfer and to devote attention to the process of holding on to the experiences gained in art therapy.

Transfer of the experience in art therapy to situations outside of therapy can be encouraged by actively asking for recognition, by actively investigating in the therapy the situation outside the therapy, and by using work forms, rituals and special interventions aimed at transfer. In a multidisciplinary treatment team, transfer can be promoted by using a consistent and shared framework between the different aspects of treatment, by the different aspects working together and by involving the client's environment in the treatment.

References

Bateman, A. W., & Fonagy, P. (2006). *Mentalization-based treatment for borderline personality disorder: A practical guide*. Oxford: Oxford University Press.

Berne, E. (1961). *Transactional analysis in psychotherapy*. New York: Grove Press Inc.

Landelijke Stuurgroep Multidisciplinaire Richtlijn ontwikkeling in de GGZ [National Advisory Committee Regarding Multidisciplinary Guidelines for Development in Mental Healthcare]. (2008). *Multidisciplinaire Richtlijn Persoonlijkheidsstoornissen. Richtlijn voor de diagnostiek en behandeling van volwassen patiënten met een persoonlijkheidsstoornis* [Multidisciplinary guideline for personality disorders. Guideline for the diagnosis and treatment of adult patients with personality disorder]. Utrecht, The Netherlands: Trimbos Instituut.

Rhyne, J. (1970). The gestalt art experience. In J. Fagan & L. L. Shepherd (Eds.), *Gestalt therapy now: Theory techniques applications*. New York, NY: Harper & Row.

Rhyne, J. (1973a). The gestalt approach to experience, art, and art therapy. *Journal of the American Art Therapy Association, 12*(4), 237–248.

Rhyne, J. (1973b). *The gestalt art experience: Patterns that connect*. Chicago, IL: Magnolia Street Publishers.

Rhyne, J. (2001). The gestalt approach to experience, art, and art therapy. *American Journal of Art Therapy, 40*(1), 109–120.

Stuiveling, G., & Van den Bergh, H. (Eds.) (1995). *Volledige Werken van Multatuli* (25 parts) (Complete works of Multatuli) (two editions).

Young, J. E. (1994). *Cognitive therapy for personality disorders: A schema-focussed approach* (Rev. ed.). Sarasota, FL: Professional Resource Press.

Young, J. E., Klosko, J., & Weishaar, M. (2003). *Schema therapy: A practitioner's guide*. New York, NY: Guilford Press.

6

'Stop Acting Out, Experience Emotions!' Child, Adult and Parent Portrayed in Art Therapy: A Case History

6.1 A Few Years Later, Former Client Katie Describes Her Experience

'I remember exactly how it all started. During my individual talk therapy I discovered that that I wanted to give words to the feelings I have about my early years (up to age 4). You can try to find the words, but I couldn't connect, my vocabulary was just not appropriate. And so the idea was to have a number of individual art therapy sessions. In group art therapy, I had found that I felt quite comfortable with art therapy.

I am very rational and analytical, but it doesn't bring me any closer to my feelings. In art therapy, you don't use words, but you feel things, literally. It happened earlier, when we were working on the circles with the rational mind, the emotional mind and the wise mind (see Chapter 3). I was working with chalk on the emotional circle, I felt huge emotions rise in me, and I had to cry. There and then, I just wanted to leave off drawing, I wanted some attention and wanted to talk about it, but I was left on my own… The therapist told me that I could just let the feelings be there, and this time I felt, 'okay, let them be there', and that was a breakthrough.

I remember that, in the group art therapy, I mapped out my social network in the assignments I made, and used all kinds of expressive elements.

S. Haeyen, *Art Therapy and Emotion Regulation Problems*,
https://doi.org/10.1007/978-3-319-96773-8_6

It felt like I was configuring my emotions. You have an overview, take some distance, but on the other hand it is all very close and tangible. Creating something in group art therapy also helped me discover how much I enjoy working with chalk, and it gave me a gift: I am still painting!

The individual art therapy was very much focused on the small child in me, who was unsure of herself, who felt hurt, frightened, lonely and neglected. A highly emotional child. As an adult, I had no idea how to deal with that. I could feel that it was part of me, but because it was so intense, I was afraid of it. I ignored it, I didn't look the small child inside of me in the eye, I didn't hold her hand. I had developed precisely my other side, the rational side. But thanks to the art therapy, I did start to look at her. And I remember that I found it extremely intense, very emotional. But at the same time I enjoyed getting to know her. The part-time therapy had helped lay a basis for this, otherwise I couldn't have done it. As an adult, I understand exactly where she is, how it all happened and how perfectly legitimate it is that she feels the way she does, and everything else about her.

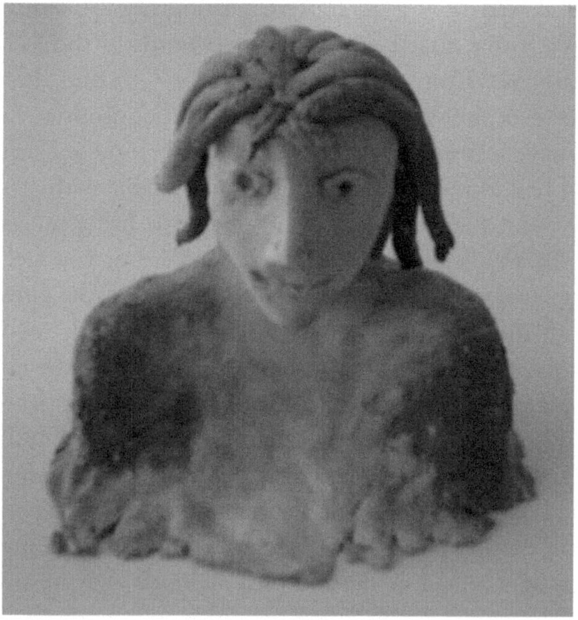

Fig. 6.1 Adult position

The first figure I made (Fig. 6.1) shows the adult position. Broad shoulders, they bear a lot of weight, I took a lot of responsibility, and those poor shoulders really hurt. The red clay on the shoulders shows my pain, makes it visible. The therapist pointed out that the figure was only a head and shoulders (actually, I hadn't really noticed) and that this perhaps showed how important the head and shoulders were, that it was a link to being very rational and analytical. I recognised that completely!

The figure of the small girl seated (Fig. 6.2) portrays very nicely how I felt when I was about seven. I even described it (as homework for in between the sessions, we were asked to write a story to go with the figure we had made): '*She feels completely lost and alone...*' Sunk in thought, she is sitting against a tree. That was then. '*The only thing I have in this whole wide world is myself*', I wrote. I felt excluded, I was not part of the family, I was different...

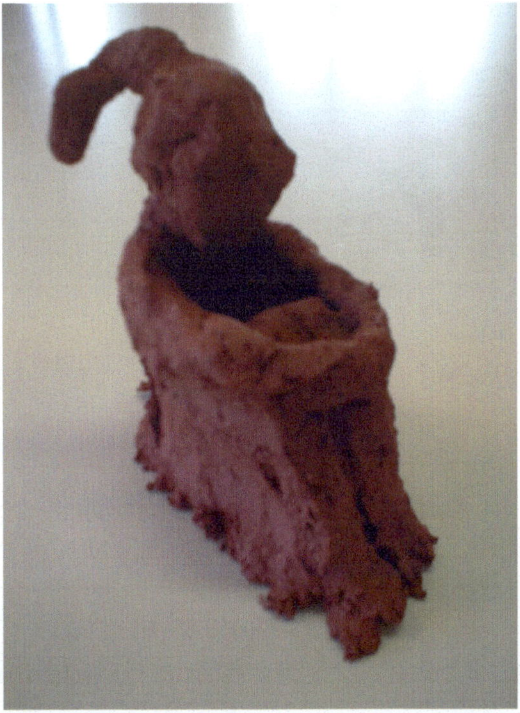

Fig. 6.2 The small girl

The writing assignment for the art therapy started out like a fictional story in the third person but it soon turned into a story about me. Still, it was nice to start out with a fantasy. Otherwise things go much too fast, everything becomes very confrontational. In the end, it was a story about a symbolic trip, a search for inner peace.

> …maybe, just maybe, there will be a day when all that changes. Maybe, just maybe, she will belong. Then maybe there will be room for people to see how kind and loyal she is.

The next question was what I, or what the child, needed. That was when I made the figure with the blanket around her (Fig. 6.3). Warmth, that is what I need, what she (the small child) needs, a warm blanket. How can you do that, how can you take care of that small, vulnerable part of yourself? Warmth was very important to me, and it still is. Someone else might say, she needs to play, but as for me, I need warmth.

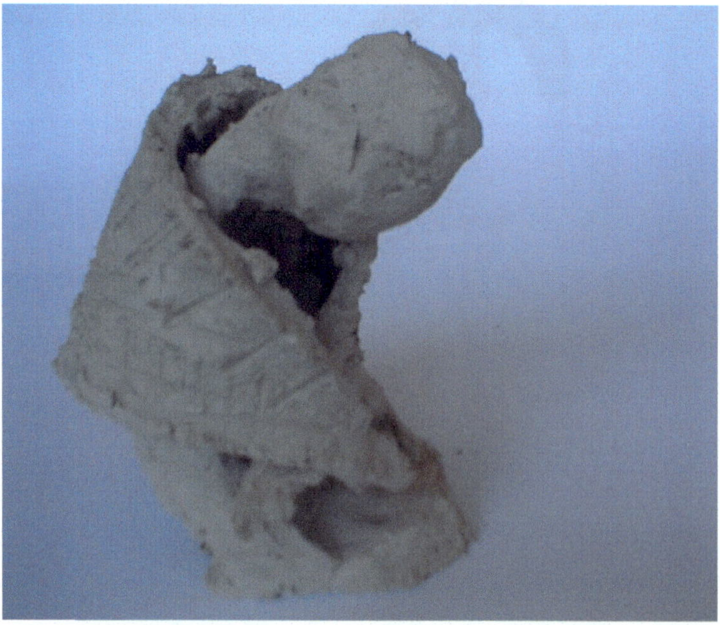

Fig. 6.3 The warm blanket

Then I was asked to bring the adult and the child together in a single figure, to make them in some sort of relationship to each other. That was when I made the big hand cupped around the small hand (Fig. 6.4). This made me realise that as an adult, I can care for the small child in myself. This figure merged all the figures, the different positions.

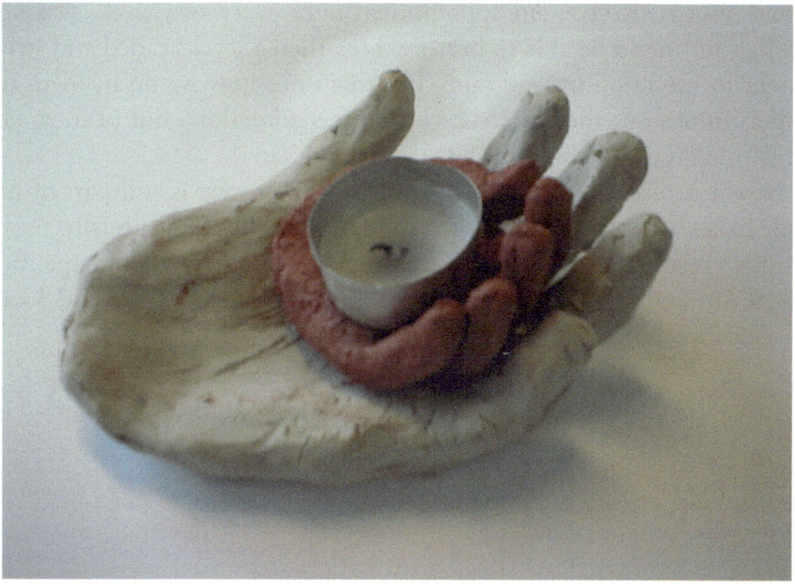

Fig. 6.4 Caring for the child in me

I used to expect others to validate me. Now I can more easily reassure myself that I am kind and loyal, even though it's a thin veneer. Still, I am becoming more stable in this respect and I'm more able to comfort myself. Now I can say to that small, vulnerable part of myself: 'it's okay, and it's hard, I know it is'.

The core of the therapy process for me was that I learned to come in contact with the vulnerable part of myself, with my feelings that go with this, and that I have started to care for that part of me. I decided to stop obsessing, stop acting out and live my life which means: experience my emotions!

This process becomes real in the way I can now get along with myself. I used to have a lot ways to feel sorry for myself; thinking worrying, I would feel strange, alienated from myself, afraid I would go crazy and lose control, and desperately trying to keep the small child or my own emotional and vulnerable side far away from me. But my emotional side presented itself after all, in my feeling sorry for myself. Before I started therapy I felt I could not go on, I couldn't hold out any longer, I no longer wanted to live. An appointment once every two weeks was not enough for me to be able to bear my life. Then a level-headed and strict parent in me stood up and said: 'But that's not how we do it, there are opportunities out there, maybe you can get something out of it, so get on with it! You can always decide to drop out later!'

Now I realise that the core of this therapy process is still part of me and, in some way or other, probably always will be. Especially in an intimate relationship, it can surface again and suddenly loom large. But now I know this, now I can more easily allow these feelings and I can care for myself better'.

7

People Diagnosed with Personality Disorders in Art Therapy: What Is the Scientific Evidence? Effectiveness of Art Therapy in Personality Disorders

7.1 Introduction

This chapter recounts the results of an extensive literature study of the effects of art therapy on personality disorders. It is in part an adapted and expanded version of the text on art therapies in the Dutch multidisciplinary guideline for personality disorders (Landelijke Stuurgroep Multidisciplinaire Richtlijn ontwikkeling in de GGZ, 2008) and the care standard for personality disorders (Zorgstandaard Persoonlijkheidsstoornissen Trimbos Instituut, 2017). The text also makes use of my PhD thesis on the effects of art therapy (Haeyen, 2018).

An evidence-based guideline or care standard contains recommendations and practical instructions to support daily practice. Such documents are based on the results of scientific research (literature) and subsequent opinion formation (experience/opinions of experts and clients) aimed at specifying what constitutes good professional conduct (CBO, 2007). For classifying evidentiary value, use was made of the classification of the Dutch healthcare quality institute CBO (see Table 7.1).

S. Haeyen, *Art Therapy and Emotion Regulation Problems*,
https://doi.org/10.1007/978-3-319-96773-8_7

Table 7.1 Classification of methodological quality of individual studies

	Intervention	Diagnostic accuracy of study
A1	Systematic review of at least two studies conducted independently of each other at A2 level	
A2	Randomised double-blind comparative clinical study of good quality and sufficient scope	Study compared to a reference test (a gold standard test), with cut-off values defined in advance and independent assessment of the results of the test and the gold standard, involving a sufficiently large series of patients all of whom were given both index test and reference test
B	Comparative study, but not with all the characteristics named under A2 (this includes patient-control study, cohort study)	Study compared to a reference test, but not with all characteristics named under A2
C	Non-comparative study (only groups of case studies according to work group on guidelines for personality disorders)	
D	Expert opinions	

Source CBO (2007)

7.2 Art Therapy in Personality Disorders in Present Practice

The object of art therapy is to set in motion change, development and acceptance processes by making expressive works. The starting point of art therapy is that the psychiatric issues can be observed in what a client does, and that these acts and therefore these experiences can be influenced in a positive direction. The treatment uses a methodical approach to attain individual objectives of change and acceptance, measured in emotional, social, behavioural, cognitive, neurological and/or physical terms (LOO VTB, 2016).

An art therapist uses interventions in the context of the expressive work. Art therapy has an important experiential, action-directed and/or creative quality. Use is made of a wide range of materials, tools and assignments that may be highly structured or highly unstructured, for example. During the process, clients acquire physical, sensorial, emotional and cognitive experiences. Emotions, feelings, thoughts and behavioural patterns that come forward in the process of making the works, playing music or completing exercises offer points of reference for reflection and communication, impulse and emotion regulation; addressing patterns in feeling, thinking and acting; and practising new roles, new skills and behavioural change. What sets art therapy apart is the fact that the works made are concrete. A client can let go of a work, put it aside, look at it again later and experience what it is like to do things differently for a change. Many clients experience art therapy as a direct route to deeper feelings. It confronts them with patterns of thinking, feeling and acting in a relatively safe situation (LOO VTB, 2016).

Nearly all treatment programmes for personality disorders work with one or more art therapists. Art therapy is among the treatment options for clients; it is included in treatment modules and programmes, often in an interrelated and shared framework. It can be given in both groups and individually. In group therapy, the focus is on interaction between the group members or on personal support to an individual in the group.

7.3 Search History

The following databases for literature on art therapy were consulted: Google Scholar, Web of Science, CINAHL, ERIC, PubMed/MEDLINE, ScienceDirect, Wiley Online Library, Embase, PsycINFO en Cochrane Library, using keywords. Keywords were 'art' or 'art therapy', in relation to personality disorders, personality, in Dutch and in English. After that, to narrow the search area, we added the keywords 'cluster A', 'cluster B', 'cluster C' and the various personality disorders, combining them in various ways with the earlier search terms. We also used professional journals, subject-related databases, manuals, modules and descriptions of studies. This literature was supplemented by descriptive literature and a panel discussion by creative therapists (Haeyen, 2005). The search was delimited by the following terms: non-forensic, age 18 and up, up to and including 2017 and language regions Dutch, English and German.

7.4 Foundations of Art Therapy Diagnostics in Personality Disorders

Art therapists investigate in dialogue with clients what problems they encounter in practice (on aspects such as planning, concentration and impulse control) and in the way clients express themselves in visual art. They are able to recognise disorders in clients' art therapy activity and in their products, and to create a climate in which together they can reach agreement at the client's level as to the meaning of the work. In addition to understanding the issues, art therapists provide information about how objectives can be attained and under what conditions. This is often not in line with a protocol, but according to experts, the method contributes to diagnosing and setting indications for art therapy for clients who are very much rationally or verbally inclined, as well as for clients who have difficulty expressing themselves verbally. This is supported by the experience and opinions of art therapists who work with clients with personality disorders as expressed in a panel discussion (Haeyen, 2005). In practice, multidisciplinary observation programmes often include art therapy. The observations that arise from this make a highly regarded contribution to diagnosing clients with personality disorder and provide information on indications for art therapy. This is the opinion of experts and so it comes under level D. A study of art therapy observation is recommended.

An art therapeutic instrument geared to (among other things) personality disorder is the Diagnostic Drawing Series (DDS). This is a diagnostic drawing test (Cohen & Mills, 2016) based on the Diagnostic and Statistical Manual of Mental Disorders (DSM; American Psychiatric Association, 2013). This test utilises an objective structural analysis of three drawings made by the client (Cohen, Hammer, & Singer, 1988). The first drawing is one of the client's choice; for the second drawing, the client is asked to draw a tree and in the third drawing, to express his or her own feelings using lines, shapes and colours. The material used is pastels in various colours. The drawings are scored on structural characteristics by an art therapist trained in the methodology. Art therapists use the DDS to compile a quick profile of a client.

The DDS offers information about how a client deals with various degrees of structure, with a question about feelings and a reaction to the task. A treatment indication can be determined on the basis of the client's motivation, willingness or ability to reflect on emotions and need for expression in this regard.

Research has shown that the diagnosis of a personality disorder can be confirmed on the basis of the drawings. A group of clients ($N=32$) diagnosed with a borderline personality disorder was scored using a blind procedure on forty image characteristics and compared with other diagnostic groups. This yielded a diagnostic profile on the basis of drawings indicative of a borderline personality disorder. In the second drawing, that of a tree, these clients exhibited disintegration as well as extravagant use of space (67–99%). Other characteristics were enclosure, mixing colours and abstract design in the third drawing (where clients were asked to express their feelings) (Mills, 1989). The instrument is described in detail in an instruction manual. Research of the degree of agreement in scoring the drawings by a number of art therapists on the standardised score list for the DDS shows that this scale has sufficient inter-rater reliability (Cohen's kappa = 0.567): 84.2% of the items were scored similarly (Fowler & Ardon, 2002). Other studies showed even higher outcomes (Mills, Cohen, & Meneses, 1993). This, a large-scale level C study, leaves little room for interpretation. The instrument is extensively described in a manual with a tutorial. There is a clearly described control group.

With regard to art therapy diagnosis of personality disorders, the conclusion is that the DDS, administered by an art therapist trained in its use, gives an indication of a diagnosis of the borderline personality disorder. The DDS also offers treatment indications for art therapy. Observation in art therapy contributes to the diagnosis and to indications for art therapy for clients with personality disorders (level D). Other considerations in this regard are that the DDS has only partial relevance for art therapy in personality disorders because it cannot yet score all the personality disorders to be distinguished. Further research to distinguish all personality disorders is recommended.

7.5 Foundations of Art Therapy Treatment in Personality Disorders

Many treatment programmes that proved effective comprise individual and/or group forms of art therapy (Bateman & Fonagy, 1999, 2004a, 2004b; Karterud & Urnes, 2004; Wilberg, Karterud, Urnes, Pedersen, & Friis, 1998). The trouble with these studies is that the contribution of art therapy to the treatment effects was not studied separately. Art therapy is often given as one aspect of a broader treatment programme. This makes it difficult to determine the effect of art therapy on its own. Bateman and Fonagy (2004a) write that the object of art therapy in part-time programmes is to offer an alternative way of promoting mentalisation in clients. The use of visual art allows what is internalised in clients to be expressed externally so that it can be verbalised from a distance and from a different perspective using the medium. Experiences and feelings are placed outside the person to facilitate explicit mentalisation. According to the authors, the experience of clients has been that this makes feelings manageable and better understood in the relatively safe (less anxiety-evoking) environment of art therapy. In clinical practice, often part of a programme is devoted to art therapy, and this policy is supported by the entire treatment staff in many institutions.

Art therapy is often part of the treatment programme for people diagnosed with personality disorders because both therapists and clients believe that it makes an important contribution to the outcome of treatment. Scientific evidence of this is, however, currently weak at best. Many currently available studies are mostly limited in sample size and quality and they seem promising at best. Art therapy needs further development and its quality could benefit from a better substantiation.

In this chapter, a link is made between the problems of clients with personality disorder and the characteristics of art therapy (art process, art product and interaction) based on literature and expert opinions. After that, the existing quantitative empirical evidence is briefly summarised.

7.5.1 Expert Opinions, Level D

Based on many descriptions of experts, it is easy to make a link between art therapy and the main problems of people with personality disorders (emotion regulation, self-regulation, enduring and inflexible patterns of cognitions, emotions and behaviours as well as impairments of interpersonal functioning—empathy or intimacy). The art therapy mechanisms seem to be well suited to the personality disorders. The following descriptions of art therapy (what it does and how it works) for personality disorder are based on expert opinions, clinical expertise and client preferences, often described in single case studies. This evidence on art therapy should therefore be qualified as the lowest level in the evidence-based pyramid, level D (CBO, 2007).

Emotional Regulation Problems

Clients diagnosed with a personality disorder often have trouble experiencing and dealing with emotions. The art therapy process offers room for exploration and experiencing emotions and inner conflicts. Feelings or themes that are difficult to process or to handle can be explored without being directly expressed in words, as is described in many handbooks on art therapy (e.g. Malchiodi, 2012; Moschini, 2005; Schweizer et al., 2009). This can help personality disorder clients to recognise these often conflicting emotions and to find a more constructive way of dealing with them. Integration of conflicting emotions can be pursued through the art work (Eisdell, 2005; Haeyen, 2007, 2011a, 2011b; Simon, 2005). Working experientially with art materials often provides a trigger to activate emotions (Keulen-de Vos, 2013; Lyshak-Stelzer, Singer, St. John, & Chemtob, 2007; Pifalo, 2006; Schouten, De Niet, Knipscheer, Kleber, & Hutschemaekers, 2014).

This is also important in traumas, particularly childhood traumas, which are often seen in clients with personality disorder (Ingenhoven, van Reekum, van Luyn, & Luyten 2012). Difficult or conflicting emotions are often avoided by personality disorder clients because they are so hard to handle. In the art therapy process (including sensory and affective perception and reflection), clients learn to undergo, recognise, process and possibly accept difficult emotions or themes (e.g. Haeyen, 2011b; Rankanen, 2016; Rubin, 2001).

The art product is concrete and tangible and may mirror the affective experience of personality disorder clients, their emotions, inner conflicts and identity. This can have a confirming effect, but can also be confrontational. For example, for someone diagnosed with a personality disorder, this may mean that the art work shows that their anger is stronger than acknowledged. The art products of people diagnosed with a personality disorder often show inner conflicts or fragmentation of the self. People diagnosed with a personality disorder often merge or fuse with their emotions and, as a result, this engulfs them, frequently leading to avoidance, suppression or diversion. This makes it more difficult for them to take a more distant perspective, and the art product can then be of help. The art product is a visible representation of their emotions. Because it shows emotions in externalised form, they can literally stand at a distance from these emotions and be 'forced' to take a stance on them, to relate to the emotions. This is described in descriptive literature and in case studies (e.g. McMurray & Schwarz-Mirman, 2001; Neumann, 2001; Toles, 1998). The art product can stimulate emotional perception (thus 'defusing' from emotions (Hayes, 2000) as opposed to merging or fusing with them), self-insight and a more observant or sometimes also more down-to-earth perspective. The art product can offer a bridge for communication, especially when fear or resistance is high (e.g. Lefevre, 2004; Moschini, 2005).

The interaction component consists of stimulating self-reflection when discussing the art work with the therapist. Personality disorder clients often get caught up in direct interactions with others, and because the art work is used as an extra pillar in the therapeutic situation, this can make interaction less direct and therefore less threatening. Transference between therapist and client is then diluted because transference also goes to the art media and art product (Gussak & Rosal, 2016; Malchiodi, 2012). Interaction related to the art process and art product can be direct as well as indirect. Emotions can be expressed in the art work without direct communication about these emotions to the therapist. The therapist can witness expressed emotional content without words or use indirect interventions to support expression (Daszkowski, 2004; Schweizer et al., 2009). Direct communication with the therapist and others is used to improve clients' understanding and handling of their own emotions.

Self-regulation Problems

Personality disorder clients often suffer from weakened autonomy and an unstable, diffuse or negative self-image. In the art process, the personality disorder client is responsible for the creation of the art product, and this asks for self-management or self-direction. Very often the art assignment of the therapist is so broadly formulated that clients themselves can determine what the product will look like. While making the art product, the personality disorder client has an internal dialogue and can experience autonomy. In the art process, choices and considerations are crucial. Experiencing more self-management or self-direction and awareness of your own choices helps strengthen or improve the sense of self, of individuality, self-awareness and self-image. This is supported by many studies and descriptive literature (e.g. Czamanski-Cohen & Weihs, 2016; Gatta, Gallo, & Vianello, 2014; Haeyen, 2007, 2011a, 2011b; Malchiodi, 2012; Neumann, 2001).

The actual art product shows the client who they are, both by the content of the image and by its formal image characteristics, as many experts agree (e.g. Gussak & Rosal, 2016; Springham, Findlay, Woods, & Harris, 2012). 'What you make is how you are'. The content of the art product is a mirror of the client's characteristics. People diagnosed with a personality disorder often experience a range emotional states (modes) in themselves and it can be very difficult to get them into alignment, making it difficult to choose a clear personal direction. The art product often shows different, conflicting sides of the person, as various authors have pointed out over the years, from the early 1980s up to the present (e.g. Haeyen, 2007; Jádi & Trixler, 1980; Rankanen, 2016). On the basis of one or several products, dialogues between these different sides can be stimulated, e.g. between the mild and the critical self. Exploring these states can eventually contribute to a less diffuse, more stable self, more self-compassion and positive self-esteem. If the art product reflects little or nothing of the client, strengthening this aspect can be the focus of work in the next art process.

In the interaction while jointly viewing the art product, focused on self-regulation problems, emphasis is on investigating and discovering the person's identity and what personal direction he or she wants to follow. The discussion of the art work is then about identity, authenticity and self-image.

Enduring and Inflexible Patterns of Cognitions, Emotions and Behaviours

Personality disorder clients have enduring and inflexible intrapersonal patterns of cognitions, emotions and behaviours that lead to significant distress or impairments, with an impact on a broad range of personal situations (APA, 2013; WHO, 2015). In the art process, fixed patterns of cognitions, emotions and behaviours as well as the way a client interacts with the art media (e.g. controlled perfectionist, impulsive or affective behaviour) are visible, according to many authors (e.g. Hinz, 2009; Schweizer et al., 2009). Alternative behaviours can be practised (e.g. from rationally stuck behaviour to more spontaneous, less controlled behaviour or from impulsive to more thoughtful). The art process can be then seen as a playing or practice field with room for experimentation. If the aim is changing enduring and inflexible patterns, emphasis is on the art process itself, on interaction and less on the actual product. In the creative process, choices are made, artistic challenges are dealt with and improvisation is often needed. This process requires fine-tuning, greater flexibility, being more constructive. Practice can lead to improvement in problem-solving skills, as well as to moving away from fixed patterns (Gussak & Rosal, 2016; Haeyen, 2007, 2015; Hinz, 2009). This would encourage personality disorder clients to cope better with personal problems in various areas of life. Art assignments, art techniques, imagination and play are used by the art therapist to make patterns visible, and then to offer challenges to induce behavioural change, as described in handbooks (e.g. Gunther, Blokland-Vos, Van Mook, & Molenaar, 2009; Van Vreeswijk, Broersen, Bloo, & Haeyen, 2012). In art therapy, the threshold to practising and playing may be lowered because challenges are offered within a safe and indirect situation with varying degrees of safety and challenges built in by the art therapist (Smeijsters, 2008). Successful experiences in making art work can encourage clients to change their feelings and thoughts; for example, 'I'm not good at anything' can be changed by experiences of success in art works to 'I can do this!' (Schnetz, 2005; Wilkinson & Chilton, 2013).

In the interaction based on the art process and art product, client and therapist look back and evaluate the concrete work process: how are patterns perceived, where are inconsistencies and where are possibilities for development (e.g. affective handling of materials involved in the art process while rationally taking more distance in the communication afterwards). The discussion of observed patterns may be about their origin, function or meaning, the desired direction to be taken or what first concrete step could lead to change.

Impairments in Interpersonal Functioning (Empathy or Intimacy)

Personality disorder clients also have problematic social patterns that lead to impairments in interpersonal functioning (empathy or intimacy) (APA, 2013; WHO, 2015). The art process can be used as a social playing or practice field; making art works then becomes a social situation in which interaction with other clients takes place via the art work, as described in several books on art therapy (Gussak & Rosal, 2016; Schweizer et al., 2009). Art therapy can then become focused on practising effective behaviour in collaboration with others (practising, for example, asking for what you need, saying no and dealing with conflicts). Group-focused art therapy may provide experiences with contact, interpersonal connection, reciprocity, play and/or autonomy.

The art product always shows traces of how interaction with others took place. Then, interaction is based in part on interpersonal functioning. Personality disorder clients may experience cognitive distortions, and evaluating the concrete process can then offer a form of reality testing. Mentalisation is also often difficult for personality disorder clients. It can be actively practised in the interaction with other participants as well as in the communication on the art work itself and the art experiences (Bateman & Fonagy, 2004a, 2004b; Springham et al., 2012; Verfaille, 2016). Improved mentalising contributes to a better understanding by personality disorder clients of themselves and others in interaction (empathy). A better understanding of different perspectives in the interpersonal functioning may also contribute to more stable relationships or to better interpersonal functioning.

7.5.2 Non-comparative Research, Level C

A total of eight non-comparative research studies were found (**level C**; CBO, 2007*)* which will be described in the order of the year of publication, from most recent to older.

Using a pre-/post-test study involving psychodynamic art therapy with 17 personality disorder clients, Eren et al. (2014) conclude that group art therapy contributes to improving global functioning in clients with personality disorders and poor treatment adherence.

Gatta et al. (2014) describe the effects of group art therapy in the setting of a residential rehabilitation centre for adolescents with personality disorders ($N = 9$). Although limitations of this study are the lack of a control group and the small sample, it provides some indications that, as part of a compulsory stay in a residential rehabilitation centre, group art therapy could have an added, aggregating value, helping the adolescents to combat the sense of solitude and self-centred isolation.

The study by Springham et al. (2012) concerns a mentalisation-based treatment programme for borderline personality disorder (B personality disorder) ($N = 6$), with an art therapy group as one of the programme's three components. This study combines quantitative and qualitative methods in a naturalistic practice setting. Evaluation shows positive results including increases in distress tolerance, lowered service use and two participants no longer meeting criteria for the B personality disorder diagnosis. The study suggests that in anchoring mental content in an externalised form, art therapy offers the flexibility to slow down the process of explicit mentalisation to a manageable pace. Limitations of this study are again the small sample size, the lack of a control group and the qualitative element being represented by a single case.

In a quantitative study by Haeyen (2011a), clients diagnosed with personality disorder cluster B and C ($N=34$) evaluated art therapy by answering the question: 'How much benefit did you gain from art therapy?' on a five-point Likert scale (1 = not; 2 = little; 3 = slightly; 4 = rather much; and 5 = much), with a mean score of 4. The goals worked on in art therapy were also evaluated. The goals that clients found were most often targeted by art therapy are 'expression of emotions', 'a more clear and stable self-image' and 'recognising, understanding and changing patterns in feelings, behaviours and thoughts'.

In a qualitative study by Haeyen, Van Hooren and Hutschemaekers (2015), clients with cluster B and C personality disorders ($N=29$) were interviewed, both individually and in a focus group. The basis for the interviews was a topic list based on literature study and a negative case. Data were collected and analysed with the Grounded Theory approach so as to form concepts and coherent categories. The results were summarised and integrated into a model consisting of five effect categories: (1) perception; (2) personal integration; (3) emotion and impulse regulation; (4) behavioural change; and (5) insight and understanding. Improved perception means experiencing the here and now, and was regarded as the basis on which the other therapeutic effects could develop. The effects included a more complete experience of self, greater balance in managing emotions and impulses, acceptance, developing and internalising other behaviour towards self and others and a better understanding of self and others. The analyses show that, compared to verbal therapy, clients experience art therapy as an experiential treatment with a complementary quality in addition to verbal therapy and as a more direct way to gain access to emotions. They attributed this to the appeal made by visual materials and to creating visual art in response to physical sensations and emotional responses. Clients declared that art therapy confronted them with themselves and their own patterns in feelings, thoughts and behaviour, reaching beyond a conscious, rational level and leading to a stronger emotional awareness. Art therapy came forward as well suited and closely connected to the core problems of people diagnosed with personality disorder; it offers a specific way to become more aware of emotions and it contributes to constructive emotion regulation.

In a small study ($N=5$), Franks and Whitaker (2007) report the results of a combined 9-month treatment programme of an art psychotherapy group alongside individual verbal psychotherapy sessions for personality disorder clients. The authors conclude that the results from the outcome measures suggest that the combination of treatments is effective, with benefits sustained over time, measured in an 8-month follow-up ($n=3$). However, given the very small sample and the possible bias (intervention not sufficiently isolated), it is not possible to generalise these results.

Another study by Haeyen (2007) reports the experiences using a one-session art therapy imagination assignment with a focus on schema modes of 48 clients diagnosed with a personality disorder cluster B/C; this study mentions effects such as self-insight and own patterns, more contact with emotions, improved emotion regulation and a corrective experience.

Lastly, Haeyen, Kleijberg and Hinz (2017) report on a thematic analysis of emotion regulation from client and art therapist perspectives ($N=11$; 8 clients and 3 art therapists) in art therapy. The target group was clients diagnosed with personality disorders cluster B/C. This qualitative study investigated the perceived effect. The study sought an explanation of the causal relationship between art therapy and the positive effects found in an earlier randomised controlled trial (RCT) (Haeyen, Van Hooren, Van der Veld, & Hutschemaekers, 2017a). In-depth interviews were held to collect data and thematic analysis was used to analyse the data and to generate and interpret themes. The results showed that, with targeted use of visual art assignments and materials plus a personally chosen approach to expressive processes on the part of the client, linked to the Expressive Therapies Continuum (Hinz, 2009), clients experienced emotions, portrayed them and shared their experiences. Often, these were emotions that clients had not been willing or able to see, or of which they had been less aware. The therapeutic effects were explained by the combination of specific factors in art therapy. These factors acted as triggers, helping clients to understand themselves better and to regulate their internal representations/images and emotions. The results highlight the fact that art therapy encourages awareness in the here and now and stimulates emotional processes through the interaction with materials.

All these non-comparative studies suggest effects of art therapy in clients with personality disorders. This suggestion fits well with what has been described above that art therapy is a means by which to come in contact with your own problems (aimed at aspects such as improved emotion regulation, a clearer and more stable self-image or increased distress tolerance) and that art therapy may well have added value.

7.5.3 Non-randomised Cohort Studies, Client-Control Studies, Level B

Only three studies report evidence on **level B** (CBO, 2007). However, all three were of moderate-to-weak quality, were too small-scale and/or were not always randomised. Firstly, Karterud and Pedersen (2004) report on components of a group-oriented, short-term day care programme for treatment of personality disorders ($N=319$). Most clients had a personality disorder (86%), mostly avoidant or borderline personality disorder. Treatment was evaluated by asking the question: 'how much benefit did you gain from therapy x?' The benefit gained by the art therapy group was scored significantly higher ($p<0.001$) than that of all other groups, and the art therapy group score correlated significantly ($p=0.005$) with the overall benefits of the programme. The multiple regression analysis also indicated a stronger effect in the art therapy group ($b=0.17$; $p=0.008$). Moreover, the more severely disturbed clients seemed to favour the pretend mode of the group art therapy. Referring to the work of Bateman and Fonagy (2006), the authors proposed that the group art therapy 'appeared to be a safe method of exploring the mind in the presence of mentalising self-objects' (Karterud & Pederson, 2004), and that the art therapy group ought to be a core element in the therapeutic programme for clients with personality disorders.

The second study, a pilot study conducted by Van den Broek, Keulen-de Vos and Bernstein (2011) ($N = 10$), focused on the extent to which schema-focused therapy (SFT) and drama, music and art therapies were able to provoke schema modes in forensic clients with a cluster B personality disorder. SFT was compared with treatment as usual (TAU) (i.e. cognitive behavioural therapy) and art therapies were compared to psychotherapy. The comparison of psychotherapy to art therapies showed a significant effect in relation to healthy modes ($d = 0.80$). Clients reported more healthy modes in art therapy groups than in psychotherapy ($T = 7.00$; $p < 0.05$). Art therapy that is part of TAU came forward as the most effective form of intervention. The conclusion is that art therapy is probably effective in provoking experiences and feelings (mental states) and promoting a healthy adult attitude to these feelings and experiences.

The last of the three studies concerned a relatively old randomised controlled study by Green, Wehling and Talsky (1987) in which art therapy was compared with TAU in a population of chronic psychiatric clients with cluster A and cluster B personality disorders in some of the cases ($N = 28$). Compared to clients receiving TAU, the clients in the art therapy condition (10 weeks) with a supportive, structured and reality-oriented approach showed improvement on measures of self-esteem and social contact. However, the target group of this study was broader than clients with personality disorders.

7.5.4 Randomised Controlled Trials and Systematic Reviews, Level A

The results of the search did not include a systematic review (meta-analysis) or randomised double-blind controlled trials. One study (Haeyen et al., 2017a) was a RCT of sufficient size (a limit of ≥ 20 subjects, set by Lebwohl, Heymann, Berth-Jones and Coulson (2010), and consistency (CBO, 2007). This effect study was quantitative, with a strong causal evidential value and an experimental set-up and was carried out in practice in the client group referred to, with a follow-up.

Haeyen et al. conducted a RCT based on a systematically developed art therapy intervention protocol. The object of this RCT was to evaluate the effects of the art therapy intervention developed for people diagnosed with personality disorder. A total of 74 adult participants diagnosed with a cluster B or C personality disorder (SCID-II) were divided at random into (1) a weekly art therapy group (11/2 hours, 10 weeks) and (2) a waiting list group. The Outcome Questionnaire 45 (OQ45), Acceptance and Action Questionnaire-II (AAQ-II) and Schema Mode Inventory (SMI) were administered at baseline, post-test (10 weeks after baseline) and follow-up (5 weeks after post-test). Seventy-five clients completed the research protocol. Treatment integrity was monitored during implementation. Compared to the clients in the waiting list group, clients who received the protocolled art therapy intervention showed a decrease in personality disorder pathology such as maladaptive schema modes (less impulsiveness, detachment, vulnerability and punitive behaviour) and avoidance of experiences (more acceptance of unpleasant inner experiences, such as thoughts, feelings and physical sensations). These clients in the experimental group also showed improved mental health at symptom level as well as adaptive schema modes (pleasant feelings, spontaneity and self-regulation). The effect sizes were large to very large. These effect sizes of the change in the outcomes indicate a substantial improvement in mental health after the intervention. The results were the same as or more pronounced than in other studies among the same target group: the same specific population of clients with a cluster B or C personality disorder or with borderline personality disorder only. The interventions consisted of outpatient treatment programmes of the same duration (three months) and intensity as weekly sessions. In conclusion, the results of this RCT show the potential of art therapy as an effective treatment option and the effectiveness of art therapy in itself. Art therapy not only reduced personality disorder pathology and maladaptive modes, but also helped clients to develop adaptive positive modes, indicating better positive mental health and self-regulation.

In the second quantitative study (Haeyen, Van Hooren, Van der Veld, & Hutschemaekers, 2017b), the data from the RCT were analysed again, and five questionnaires (AAQ-II, Dutch Mental Health Continuum-Short Form (MHC-SF), Mindful Attention Awareness Scale (MAAS), SMI-II adaptive—maladaptive scales and two subscales from OQ45) were divided into two domains, positive mental health and mental illness, to compare the results on these two domains of effect. The results showed very large effect sizes on outcome measures for psychological disorders as well as those for mental health. Art therapy proved to be not only a generic intervention to improve well-being and quality of life, but also a specific therapy to reduce specific symptoms. Mental health showed a strong relationship with symptoms of mental illness.

7.6 Conclusions

With regard to art therapeutic diagnosis of personality disorders, the conclusion is that the DDS, administered by an art therapist trained in its use, gives an indication of a diagnosis in relation to borderline personality disorder and treatment indications for art therapy. In order to distinguish all personality disorders, further research is recommended.

In conclusion, art therapy proved effective for people diagnosed with personality disorder: it reduced general psychological dysfunctioning as well as specific symptoms of cluster B and C personality disorders. Early maladaptive behaviour or emotional states that are typical of a personality disorder decreased (less impulsiveness, disconnection, vulnerability and punitive behaviour) and the presence of adaptive modes increased (pleasant feelings and self-regulation). Unpleasant inner thoughts, feelings and physical sensations seemed to be more readily accepted and mindful attention increased. Art therapy was effective in the domain of positive mental health but equally effective in the domain of psychological disorder. Art therapy was effective in evoking experiences and feelings (mental states) in clients with a personality disorder and had a positive effect on emotion regulation.

Clients indicated that art therapy had taught them to deal with difficult emotions, to take action, make choices and express their emotions. It made it possible to restore emotional contact with experiences.

Art therapy resulted in integration of conflicting emotions at an intra-psychological level. Clients also indicated that art therapy helped them to develop their internal dialogue, at their own pace, as well as expression and self-reflection based on the process and the expressive product.

This is explained in that art therapy has a different dynamic to verbal therapy; it is more gradual, with relatively greater concentration on the self and more undisturbed inner dialogue. In addition, personal insight and understanding are gained in relation to their patterns, and this provides input for behavioural change. Compared to the more cognitive verbal therapies, clients often experience art therapy as a better therapeutic way of exploring dysfunctional patterns. More systematic research of the effects and operational mechanisms of art therapy in people with personality disorder is needed.

A few further considerations also play a role. Firstly, it is important to remember that, in many cases, traumas are involved (e.g. sexual traumas, neglect and abuse) in this target group. Despite the fact that it was not the primary focus in this search, it comes forward in various that art therapy can make a positive contribution to the treatment of both personality disorder and traumas (Schouten et al., 2014), in order to arrive at acceptance and/or change. For eating disorders that are simultaneously present, art therapy may contribute to self-insight and a realistic self-image (Levens, 1990).

Secondly, experiential techniques have recently received more attention from verbal therapies. Experiential techniques are increasingly being included in a range of cognitive behavioural therapies (such as SFT or acceptance and commitment therapy (ACT) and are mainly used to supplement a central basis of verbal interventions. For example, Arntz (2011, 2012) claimed that when used as part of SFT, these experiential techniques held promise for therapeutic use, although he stressed the need to subject these techniques to systematic empirical evaluation so as to test their effectiveness and to unravel the underlying mechanisms of change. The results in the RCT show that art therapy is in itself powerful, and not only as a supplement to a verbal therapy.

Lastly, it is recommended to offer verbal and art therapeutic treatment in combination with a multidisciplinary treatment. Art therapy can be part of learning by experience and may be a good fit to a possible affinity of the client and can thus offer a pleasant therapeutic gateway (and one that may well be effective on this account). A shared and consistently used framework in the multidisciplinary treatment of personality disorder is important because that is precisely what has proved to be effective, rather than what theory is used (Landelijke Stuurgroup Multidisciplinaire Richtlijn in de GGZ, 2008).

References

American Psychiatric Association [APA]. (2013). *Diagnostic and statistical manual of mental disorders* (5th ed.). Washington, DC: American Psychiatric Association.

Arntz, A. (2011). Imagery rescripting for personality disorders. *Cognitive and Behavioural Practice, 18,* 466–481. https://doi.org/10.1016/j.cbpra.2011.04.006.

Arntz, A. (2012). Imagery rescripting as a therapeutic technique: Review of clinical trials, basic studies, and research agenda. *Journal of Experimental Psychopathology, 3,* 189–208. https://doi.org/10.5127/jep.024211.

Bateman, A. W., & Fonagy, P. (1999). Effectiveness of partial hospitalization in the treatment of borderline personality disorder: A randomised controlled trial. *American Journal of Psychotherapy, 156,* 1563–1569. https://doi.org/10.1176/ajp.156.10.1563.

Bateman, A. W., & Fonagy, P. (2004a). *Psychotherapy for borderline personality disorder: Mentalisation based treatment.* New York: Oxford University Press.

Bateman, A. W., & Fonagy, P. (2004b). Mentalization-based treatment of personality disorder. *Journal of Personality Disorders, 18,* 36–51. https://doi.org/10.1521/pedi.18.1.36.32772.

Bateman, A. W., & Fonagy, P. (2006). *Mentalization-based treatment for borderline personality disorder: A practical guide.* Oxford: Oxford University Press.

CBO [Kwaliteitsinstituut voor de gezondheidszorg]. (2007). *Handleiding voor werkgroepleden* [Manual for members of a work group]. Utrecht: CBO.

Cohen, B. M., & Mills, A. (2016). The Diagnostic Drawing Series (DDS) at thirty: Art therapy assessment and research. In D. Gussak & M. Rosal (Eds.), *The Wiley handbook of art therapy* (pp. 558–568). Hoboken, NJ: Wiley-Blackwell.

Cohen, B. M., Hammer, J., & Singer, S. (1988). The diagnostic drawing series: A systematic approach to art therapy evaluation and research. *The Arts in Psychotherapy, 15,* 11–21.

Czamanski-Cohen, J., & Weihs, K. (2016). The bodymind model: A platform for studying the mechanisms of change induced by art therapy. *The Arts in Psychotherapy, 51,* 63–71. https://doi.org/10.1016/j.aip.2016.08.006.

Daszkowski, A. (2004). Alles unter einem Dach: Die integrative Funktion der kunsttherapie in der stationaren Borderline-behandlung [Under the same roof: The integrated function of art therapy in the clinical treatment of borderline clients]. *Personlichkeitsstorungen Theorie und Therapie, 8*(3), 143–153.

Eisdell, N. (2005). A conversational model of art therapy. *Psychology and Psychotherapy, 78,* 1–19. https://doi.org/10.1348/147608305X40840.

Eren, N., Öğünç, N. E., Keser, V., Bıkmaz, S., Şahin, D., & Saydam, B. (2014). Psychosocial, symptomatic and diagnostic changes with long-term psychodynamic art psychotherapy for personality disorders. *The Arts in Psychotherapy, 41,* 375–385. https://doi.org/10.1016/j.aip.2014.06.004.

Fowler, J. P., & Ardon, A. M. (2002). Diagnostic drawing series and dissociative disorders: A Dutch study. *The Arts in Psychotherapy, 29,* 221–230.

Franks, M., & Whitaker, R. (2007). The image, mentalisation and group art psychotherapy. *International Journal of Art Therapy, 12,* 3–16. https://doi.org/10.1080/17454830701265188.

Gatta, M., Gallo, C., & Vianello, M. (2014). Art therapy groups for adolescents with personality disorders. *The Arts in Psychotherapy, 41,* 1–6. https://doi.org/10.1016/j.aip.2013.11.001.

Green, B. L., Wehling, C., & Talsky, G. J. (1987). Group art therapy as an adjunct to treatment for chronic outclients. *Hospital Community Psychiatry, 38,* 988–991. https://doi.org/10.1176/ps.38.9.988.

Gunther, G., Blokland-Vos, J., van Mook, C., & Molenaar, J. P. (2009). Vaktherapie binnen klinische schematherapie [Arts therapies within clinical scheme therapy]. In E. Muste, A. Weertman, & A. Claassen (Eds.), *Handboek klinische schematherapie* [Handbook on clinical scheme therapy] (pp. 99–130). Houten: Bohn Stafleu van Loghum.

Gussak, D., & Rosal, M. (Eds.). (2016). *The Wiley handbook of art therapy.* Hoboken, NJ: Wiley-Blackwell.

Haeyen, S. (2005). Panel discussion for experienced arts therapist about arts therapies in the treatment of personality disorders. *Internal document on behalf of the development of the national multi-disciplinary guideline for the treatment of personalities disorders.* Utrecht: Trimbos Instituut.

Haeyen, S. (2007). *Niet uitleven maar beleven: Beeldende therapie bij persoonlijkheidsproblematiek*. Houten: Bohn Stafleu van Loghum.

Haeyen, S. (2011a). *De verbindende kwaliteit van beeldende therapie. Effecten van beeldende therapie in de behandeling van persoonlijkheidsstoornissen*. Antwerpen: Garant.

Haeyen, S. (2011b). *Vaktherapie: De kracht van de ervaring*. In T. Ingenhoven, A. van Reekum, B. van Luyn, & P. Luyten (Eds.), *Handboek borderline persoonlijkheidsstoornis* [Borderline personality disorder handbook] (pp. 215–227). Utrecht: De Tijdstroom.

Haeyen, S. (2015). De gezonde volwassene verstevigen in beeldende therapie. In A. Claassen & S. Pol (Eds.), *Schematherapie en de gezonde volwassene: Positieve technieken uit de praktijk* (pp. 157–173). Houten: Bohn Stafleu van Loghum.

Haeyen, S. (2018). *Effects of art therapy. The case of personality disorders cluster B/C* (Dissertation manuscript). Nijmegen: Proefschriftmaken.nl.

Haeyen, S., Kleijberg, M., & Hinz, L. D. (2017). Art therapy for clients with personality disorders cluster B/C: A thematic analysis of emotion regulation from client and art therapist perspectives. *International Journal of Art Therapy*, Published online: 8 December 2017. https://doi.org/10.1080/17454832.2017.1406966.

Haeyen, S., van Hooren, S., & Hutschemaekers, G. (2015). Perceived effects of art therapy in the treatment of personality disorders, cluster B/C: A qualitative study. *The Arts in Psychotherapy, 45*, 1–10. https://doi.org/10.1016/j.aip.2015.04.005.

Haeyen, S., van Hooren, S., van der Veld, W., & Hutschemaekers, G. (2017a). Efficacy of art therapy in individuals with personality disorders cluster B/C: A randomized controlled trial. *Journal of Personality Disorders*. Advance online publication. https://doi.org/10.1521/pedi_2017_31_312.

Haeyen, S., van Hooren, S., van der veld, W., & Hutschemaekers, G. (2017b). Promoting mental health versus reducing mental illness in art therapy with clients with personality disorders: A quantitative study. *The Arts in Psychotherapy, 58*, 11–16. https://doi.org/10.1080/17454832.2017.1406966.

Hayes, S. C. (2000, June). Acceptance and commitment therapy in the treatment of experiential avoidance disorders. *Clinician's Research Digest: Supplemental Bulletin, 22*, 1–2.

Hinz, L. D. (2009). *Expressive therapies continuum: A framework for using art in therapy*. New York: Routledge.

Ingenhoven, T., van Reekum, M., van Luyn, B., & Luyten, P. (Eds.). (2012). *Handboek borderline persoonlijkheidsstoornis* [Handbook on borderline personality disorder]. Utrecht: De Tijdstroom.

Jádi, F., & Trixler, M. (1980). The use of focal model in art therapy. *Confinia psychiatry, 23,* 93–102.

Karterud, S., & Pedersen, G. (2004). Short-term day hospital treatment for personality disorders: Benefits of the therapeutic components. *Therapeutic Communities: International Journal for Therapeutic & Supportive Organisations, 25,* 43–54.

Karterud, S., & Urnes, O. (2004). Short-term day treatment programmes for cliënts with personality disorders. What is the optimal composition? *Nordic Journal of Psychiatry, 58*(3), 243–249.

Keulen-de Vos, M. E. (2013). *Emotional states, crime and violence: A schema therapy approach to the understanding and treatment of forensic clients with personality disorders* (Dissertation manuscript). Maastricht: Datawyse/ Maastricht University Press.

Landelijke Stuurgroep Multidisciplinaire Richtlijn ontwikkeling in de GGZ [National Advisory Committee Regarding Multidisciplinary Guidelines for Development in Mental Healthcare]. (2008). *Multidisciplinaire Richtlijn Persoonlijkheidsstoornissen. Richtlijn voor de diagnostiek en behandeling van volwassen patiënten met een persoonlijkheidsstoornis* [Multidisciplinary guideline for personality disorders. Guideline for the diagnosis and treatment of adult clients with personality disorder]. Utrecht: Trimbos Instituut.

Lebwohl, M., Heymann, W., Berth-Jones, J., & Coulson, I. (2010). *Treatment of skin disease—Comprehensive therapeutic strategies* (3rd ed.). New York: Saunders-Elsevier.

Lefevre, M. (2004). Finding the key: Containing and processing traumatic sexual abuse. *The Arts in Psychotherapy, 31,* 137–152. https://doi.org/10.1016/j.aip.2004.05.001.

Levens, M. (1990). Borderline aspects in eating disorders: Art therapy's contribution. *Group Analysis, 23,* 277–284. https://doi.org/10.1177/0533316490233008.

LOO VTB. (2016). *Landelijk Domeinprofiel Bacheloropleidingen Vaktherapeutische Beroepen* [National guideline regarding bachelor programmes for arts and psychomotor therapies professions]. Nijmegen: LOO VTB.

Lyshak-Stelzer, F., Singer, P., St. John, P., & Chemtob, C. (2007). Art therapy for adolescents with posttraumatic stress disorder symptoms: A pilot study. *Journal of the American Art Therapy Association, 24,* 163–169. https://doi.org/10.1080/07421656.2007.10129474.

Malchiodi, C. A. (2012). *Handbook of art therapy* (2nd ed.). New York: Guilford.
McMurray, M., & Schwarz-Mirman, O. (2001). Integration and working through in art therapy. *The Arts in Psychotherapy, 28,* 311–318. https://doi.org/10.1016/S0197-4556(01)00123-X.
Mills, A. (1989). A statistical study of the formal aspects of the DDS of borderline personality disordered clients, and its context in contemporary art therapy (Unpublished master's thesis). Concordia University, Montreal.
Mills, A., Cohen, B. M., & Meneses, J. Z. (1993). Reliability and validity tests of the diagnostic drawing series. *The Arts in Psychotherapy, 20,* 83–88.
Moschini, L. B. (2005). Part I: Defence mechanisms and the norms of behavior. In *Drawing the line, art therapy with the difficult client.* Hoboken, NJ: Wiley.
Neumann, E. (2001). Forschungsperspektiven integrativer klinischer Kunsttherapie am beispiel einer borderlineproblematik. *Musik-, tanz- und Kunsttherapie, 12,* 171–187. https://doi.org/10.1026//0933-6885.12.4.171.
Pifalo, T. (2006). Art therapy with sexually abused children and adolescents: Extended research study. *Art Therapy, 23,* 181–185. https://doi.org/10.1080/07421656.2006.10129337.
Rankanen, M. (2016). *The visible spectrum: Participants' experiences of the process and impacts of art therapy* (Dissertation manuscript). Doctoral Dissertations (141), Aalto University, Espoo, Finland.
Rubin, J. (2001). *Approaches to art therapy: Theory and technique.* New York: Routledge.
Schnetz, M. (2005). *The healing flow: Artistic expression in therapy.* London: Jessica Kingsley.
Schouten, K., De Niet, G., Knipscheer, J., Kleber, R., & Hutschemaekers, G. (2014). The effectiveness of art therapy in the treatment of traumatized adults. *Trauma, Violence, and Abuse, 16,* 220–228. https://doi.org/10.1177/1524838014555032.
Schweizer, C., Bruyn, J., Haeyen, S., Henskens, B., Rutten-Saris, M., & Visser, H. (2009). *Handboek beeldende therapie: Uit de verf* [Handbook of art therapy: Express yourself]. Houten: Bohn Stafleu van Loghum.
Simon, R. M. (2005). *Self-healing through visual and verbal art therapy.* London: Jessica Kingsley.
Smeijsters, H. (2008). *Handboek creatieve therapie* [Handbook of the arts therapies] (3rd ed.). Bussum: Coutinho.

Springham, N., Findlay, D., Woods, A., & Harris, J. (2012). How can art therapy contribute to mentalization in borderline personality disorder? *International Journal of Art Therapy, 17,* 115–129. https://doi.org/10.1080/17454832.2012.734835.

Toles, M. M. (1998). Secure-separation through secure-attachment: A 2 year single-case study involving intense therapy with a severe borderline personality disordered subject. *Dissertation Abstract Internationals: Section B: The Sciences and Engineering, 59*(3-B), 1381.

Trimbos Instituut. (2017). *Zorgstandaard persoonlijkheidsstoornissen: Kwaliteitsontwikkeling GGZ* [Care standard personality disorders: Quality development mental health care]. Utrecht: Trimbos Instituut. Concept version d.d. 23 May 2017.

Van den Broek, E., Keulen-de Vos, M., & Bernstein, D. P. (2011). Arts therapies and schema focussed therapy: A pilot study. *The Arts in Psychotherapy, 38,* 325–332. https://doi.org/10.1016/j.aip.2011.09.005.

Van Vreeswijk, M., Broersen, J., Bloo, J., & Haeyen, S. (2012). Techniques within schema therapy. In M. van Vreeswijk, J. Broersen, & M. Nadort (Eds.), *The Wiley-Blackwell handbook of schema therapy: Theory, research, and practice* (pp. 185–195). Chichester: Wiley.

Verfaille, M. (2016). *Mentalizing in arts therapies.* London: Karnac Books.

WHO [World Health Organization]. (2015). *International classification of diseases, tenth revision, clinical modification (ICD-10-CM).* Geneva: WHO.

Wilberg, T., Karterud, S., Urnes, O., Pedersen, G., & Friis, S. (1998). Outcomes of poorly functioning clients with personality disorders in a day treatment program. *Psychiatric Services, 49,* 1462–1467. https://doi.org/10.1176/ps.49.11.1462.

Wilkinson, R., & Chilton, G. (2013). Positive art therapy: Linking positive psychology to art therapy theory, practice, and research. *Art Therapy, 30,* 4–11. https://doi.org/10.1080/07421656.2013.757513.

Part II

Workbook

The workbook is organised along the lines of the skills training for the four modules constituting the dialectical behaviour therapy of Marsha Linehan: mindfulness, emotion regulation, interpersonal effectiveness and distress tolerance (Linehan in *Cognitive-behavioural treatment of borderline personality disorder.* Guildford Press, New York, NY, 1993; Linehan in *Borderline persoonlijkheidsstoornisstoornis. Handleiding voor training en therapie* [Skills training manual for treating borderline personality disorder]. Swets & Zeitlinger, Lisse, The Netherlands, 1996). This information is supplemented with a module providing an introduction to the schema-focused therapy of Jeffrey Young (Young in *Cognitive therapy for personality disorders: A schema-focused approach* (Rev. ed.). Professional Resource Press, Sarasota, FL, 1994, Young, Klosko, & Weishaar in *Schema therapy: A practitioner's guide.* Guilford Press, New York, NY, 2003) and a group of methods to be used in special situations. The introduction describes the therapeutic attitude and introduces the assignments and variations in starting and closing of sessions. It provides a product description for the whole art therapy programme for people diagnosed with a personality disorder and a summary of dialectical behaviour therapy.

Introduction

The workbook is organised along the lines of the skills training for the four modules constituting the dialectical behaviour therapy of Marsha Linehan: mindfulness, emotion regulation, interpersonal effectiveness and distress tolerance (Linehan, 1993, 1996). This information is supplemented with a module providing an introduction to the schema-focused therapy of Jeffrey Young (Young, 1994; Young, Klosko, & Weishaar, 2003) and a group of methods to be used in special situations.

The methods for special situations can be put to use, for example, when a new person joins the group, when a crisis occurs in the group or when a member of the group is leaving. Selected work forms are used on these special occasions on account of the importance attached to rituals, with a focus on developing the necessary skills.

All work forms used are tailored to use in an open group, one which clients join when they start and leave when they stop. This situation will be familiar to many therapists as it frequently occurs in practice. The clients have been diagnosed and selected during the intake for personality problems or disorders, motivation and therapeutic possibilities. This therapeutic programme therefore does not include a separate observation period. An observation module, separate from the modules here, might well be included under different circumstances.

Attention is also paid to the group dynamics, which shows that the approach is not simply skills training, but rather therapy with training elements. This differs from the Linehan skills training method (Linehan, 1993, 1996).

Each module in the workbook comprises a summary of the theory behind it, an overview of the multidisciplinary relationships in the module and a number of art therapy assignments. When working in a multidisciplinary programme, close connections with the other components of treatment are important (Bateman & Fonagy, 2006; Fonagy & Bateman, 2005). The various disciplines have described their own contribution to each module.

Using the Workbook

It is not the aim of the skills training modules to present a fixed series of assignments that must be followed. The aim is to offer a set of assignments per module, from which a selection can be made that is attuned to the individuals in the group and the group's phase of development. The degree of structure offered in a given assignment can be increased by adapting it to suit the group. These adaptations mean that the assignments presented can be transferred and used in other situations as well.

Therapeutic Attitude and Interventions

Freedom and Structure, Autonomy, Challenge and Security, Guidance

This group of clients has a high level of anxiety and, most notably, a fear of being overwhelmed by their own emotions. This means that clients must learn to deal with their emotions in a controlled manner. They must be confident that they will be able to handle the pace in cooperation with the therapist. The team members must know how to act in a crisis situation. To help these clients acquire new knowledge and skills, a calm and relaxed environment is needed; otherwise, new information cannot be adequately absorbed and processed. Calm is created by providing a safe and predictable environment: in each session, the objective, the approach and limits must be made clear to clients. Security is also created by taking utmost care in the interaction with the client: the individual objectives must be known; files must be complete; relevant information must be communicated in a timely manner to members of the team and the responsible therapist. During art therapy, therapeutic interventions and therapeutic attitude are based on a number of principles. These include considerable attention to client autonomy and letting clients take as much individual responsibility as possible within the structure of the assignment they are working on. In addition, clients must be encouraged to take risks, to practise and experiment with different types of behaviour, to acknowledge other emotions and form different thoughts.

How the Therapy Is Offered; Importance of Clarity and Transparency

Due to the high state of arousal which characterises most of these clients, they require, first and foremost, clarity and structure. Expanding their sense of control and security is therefore of primary importance and forms the basis on which they will work. This can be achieved by offering treatment with a very transparent and unambiguous structure and approach. The success of an assignment depends on how it is presented. Clarity and transparency are important for this target group. The therapist must be trustworthy, provide continuity and be open. In addition to a clear explanation of the assignments and methods to be used, it is important that the manner in which this information is presented invites clients to be active and start exploring the materials or themes to which they have been introduced.

The client needs to see the importance of the assignments, if not before working then afterwards. This does not mean that the objective of the assignment is always purposely clarified in advance. Sometimes making the client aware of the objective of an assignment before carrying it out can invalidate the experience. And sometimes asking for more explanation before carrying out an assignment is simply a way for the client to put off starting on it. At that point, this is a good reason to act first and discuss it later. Later, as the therapist, you can provide a transparent explanation for the choice of a particular assignment, if the experience itself has not already made it clear.

Respect and Validation

Respect for the client and reinforcement of all behaviour which is slightly in the right direction (even if it is only an intention) are important for the development of the client's self-respect, which has often been severely damaged. In this way, clients perceive that their difficulties have been acknowledged, and their often emotionally charged past as well.

Regulation of the Contact

The target client group is known to experience strong feelings of dependency but at the same time, a fear of losing their autonomy. This situation calls for careful regulation of the distance–closeness in contact with a client and, for example, the adoption of a friendly, generally professional attitude. Treatment should be aimed at promoting autonomy and helping the client learn, with your support, to manage his or her own problems.

The therapist should not be lured into a conflict or discussion but should turn the contact into something the client and the therapist can examine. In order to do this, limits must be made clear for expressions of aggression, forms of interaction and other matters which can undermine or threaten the therapy. It is important that the therapist does not feel personally attacked, is not guided by countertransference and can offer a good example of how to deal with difficult situations.

Negotiation
Negotiation is a basic characteristic of the therapeutic relation between client and therapist. This means that, when a client has good reasons for it, the group, or an individual in the group, can deviate from the assignment at hand. The therapist then acts as a coach, asks questions, thinks along with the client, but does not provide answers as such.

Linking Tasks to Theoretical Frameworks by Explanation and Behaviour
The therapist makes direct use of the theory that provides the starting point for each of the modules. This is done by explaining the theory, using terms from the theory, referring to the theory during interventions and encouraging clients to connect experience with theory or, in other words, frame their experience in terms of the theory in the follow-up discussion. The themes addressed in the modules provide the theoretical guideline and framework for the client's experience; these themes determine the direction of the interventions at that moment.

Tension Between Individual Needs and the Group as a Whole
It is important to recognise the tension between the structure provided at the level of the group and needs at the individual level. Individuals must have enough strength to reasonably maintain themselves within the group and the structure of the programme. Room for individual support and/or adaptation of the programme can be created if necessary.

The Assignments
The assignments and the way they are structured in this workbook have been developed and evaluated in actual practice. The 106 assignments are outlined in practical terms and hopefully offer every art therapist not only recognisable guidelines but also new ideas and practical pointers. The assignments have been gathered over a period of years, which

means that their origin is not always clear. Some assignments have been around for ages; some have been modified; some I developed myself. I hope that this provides a rich collection for others to draw from. It has certainly been the case for me.

Variations in Getting Started with Art Therapy

It is often difficult to get started after the opening, in which the therapy is attuned to the clients and their current emotional state. A warming-up exercise can sometimes provide a good introduction. It can be aimed at getting moving, making contact with the material or exploring the inner experience. A warming up is typically low-threshold and therefore particularly well suited to conducting little experiments, trying something out or just doing something which otherwise, if you gave it more significance, might create more inhibition.

Some suggestions for a warming up are:

- Take a moment to make a personal weather report, a brief sketch of your inner state at this time.
- Scribble or sketch something on the paper to show how you are feeling right now.
- A material-oriented warming up to come into contact with the material and the possibilities it offers. For example, scribbling with chalk, making a ball out of clay, mixing some paint, drawing a transition from light to dark, tearing up pieces of paper…

Variations in the Follow-Up Discussion of Works Produced

Asking clients to say something about the work they have made or the process of creating, it is not always the best way for clients to discuss the assignment. When a group has little spontaneous interaction and a low level of dynamics, you can change this by taking a different tack for the follow-up discussion. By varying your approach in the follow-up discussion, it becomes less predictable, less routine. Some options are as follows:

- Each member of the group writes down a title for each of the works made in the session. For each work, each person then reads out the title they have come up with. The maker of the work reads their own title last. The maker is asked to react to the other titles as well.

- Let the work 'speak for itself' by saying what you think it might say if it could talk. It is important to recognise here that something usually comes to mind quickly, but can then be discarded just as quickly. Emphasise that this does not have to be a justified or well-considered response; it is about the first association to come to mind. A variation is: 'Imagine that the work could produce a sound, what sound would it make?'
- Have everyone move their work one place over. Everyone now has someone else's work in front of them, and the assignment is to say something about it as if they had made it themselves. Here it is striking that a great deal can be projected into a work made by someone else, or that other clients can often more openly and directly put into words what the maker experienced in making the work.
- …

Sections of the Workbook

A product description of the art therapy module as a whole.

A brief description of dialectical behaviour therapy (Linehan, 1993, 1996).

An outline of the cycle of modules to be followed during treatment:

- Mindfulness
- Emotion regulation
- Interpersonal effectiveness
- Distress tolerance
- Introduction to Schema-Focused Therapy (Young, 1994; Young, Klosko, & Weishaar, 2003)
- This information can be supplemented with:
- Assignments for special situations (as needed)

Each module starts with a brief description of the theory. For more extensive information, the list of references (below) can be used. This is followed by an overview of the multidisciplinary relationships in the treatment to show how the disciplines have different perspectives but still work with the same theory.

In Appendix 3, three art therapeutic product descriptions can be found. These are suited to a greater or lesser degree for use with clients with personality problems, depending on the severity of the problems and any additional issues. 'Focus on self' is aimed at trauma and autonomy, followed by an eating disorders module and a module aimed at learning to express feelings.

References

Bateman, A. W., & Fonagy, P. (2006). *Mentalization-based treatment for borderline personality disorder: A practical guide.* Oxford, UK: Oxford University Press.

Fonagy, P., & Bateman, A. W. (2005). Progress in the treatment of borderline personality disorder. *British Journal of Psychiatry, 188,* 1–3. doi: https://doi.org/10.1192/bjp.bp.105.012088.

Linehan, M. M. (1993). *Cognitive-behavioural treatment of borderline personality disorder.* New York, NY: Guildford Press.

Linehan, M. M. (1996). *Borderline persoonlijkheidsstoornisstoornis. Handleiding voor training en therapie* [Skills training manual for treating borderline personality disorder]. Lisse, The Netherlands: Swets & Zeitlinger.

Young, J. (1994). *Cognitive therapy for personality disorders: A schema-focussed approach* (Rev. ed.). Sarasota, FL: Professional Resource Press.

Young, J., Klosko, J., & Weishaar, M. (2003). *Schema therapy: A practitioner's guide.* New York: Guilford Press.

Product Description

Art therapy group for people diagnosed with a personality disorder Dialectical behaviour therapy and schema-focused therapy as the basis for art therapy

Author: Suzanne Haeyen

Treatment programme: personality disorders, outpatient treatment or part-time treatment

Treatment approach: Focused, insight-oriented

Rationale	Dialectical behaviour therapy and schema-focused therapy are cognitive behaviour therapies with a broad basis, specifically developed for people with personality issues. The most important underlying assumption is that the problems involve dysregulation of emotions. In the treatment, everything is therefore aimed at teaching clients to regulate their emotions. In the Linehan art therapy group, a connection is made between the experience of the here and now and Linehan's theory The dialectic often stands out quite concretely and visibly in art therapy work as that which gives expression or tension to the work. The process of *giving shape—stepping back/ reflecting—giving new shape* corresponds to the principle of synthesis—antithesis—synthesis As they use the various work forms, clients experience a clear connection between theory and their own experience. When a Linehan art therapy group is offered in combination with Linehan skills training or a part-time programme, a fruitful joint effort can emerge and contribute to effective treatment An introductory module to acquaint clients with schema-focused therapy is included in this approach. On the basis of Young's schema theory, clients work in art therapy on giving personal shape to these and examining their thought patterns on the basis of the exercises
Indications	Clients with personality disorders or emotion regulation problems who are motivated to look at their feelings, thoughts and actions, to explore them in greater detail and who have a desire to change them
Contra-indications	If the client does not have the capacity to benefit from a group or if there is a great chance that it will not be possible to establish a working relationship, or if the client cannot function independently and does not have ongoing crises under control

(continued)

Objectives	1. Gaining insight into their own emotions, thoughts and behaviour 2. Developing a capacity to express and regulate emotions 3. Attaining a more stable self-image 4. Improving interpersonal skills 5. Improving distress tolerance skills and problem-solving capacity
Interventions	Directly connected to the art therapy work is learning to acknowledge and accept how the process of creating a work unfolds. Interventions are also aimed at eliciting change: strengthening, expanding or trying the opposite (See objective 1) Clients gain insight into their own emotions, thoughts and behaviour by reflecting on what they create during art therapy and treating it as a mirror on their own inner world. Experiencing similarities with and differences to others contributes to this process (See objective 2) Emotion regulation is addressed by giving visual expression and analysing the expression by dividing the process into giving shape to something—the product—observing—experiencing—interpreting—giving new shape (See objective 3) A more stable self-awareness is attained by clients recognising and accepting the uniqueness of their own works. Self-awareness is expanded by experiencing, discussing and analysing both the individual work and the work produced by a group Bringing the often very divergent aspects (polarities) of the person together in a single piece of work promotes a sense of unity, of wholeness (See objective 4) Interpersonal skills are practised by reacting to each other, expressing recognition and admiration and giving feedback. During the shared exercises, interpersonal interactions play a role, and clients can experiment with other behaviour

(continued)

	(See objective 5) Their work in art therapy also influences the problem-solving capacity of clients. Learning to search for new or alternative solutions is stimulated. Trying things out and allowing yourself to play with materials and possibilities are important aspects of the therapy. The capacity to distract themselves by directing their thoughts to pleasant feelings is also addressed The art therapy is subdivided into modules in which the core objectives recur: mindfulness, emotion regulation, distress tolerance skills, interpersonal effectiveness skills and schema-focused therapy. Each module is composed of a number of specific art therapy assignments which are based on the theory. Use is made, for example, of methods from Gestalt therapy and Creative Problem Solving. The methods used are experiential, aimed at observing, structuring emotionally and exploring. The therapist acts as a coach, thus placing responsibility with the client as far as possible, but provides structure at the same time
Prerequisites	A safety net must be available in case a crisis situation arises
Subtypes	This product is preferably offered in combination with a Linehan/Young skills training group or therapy group
Duration and frequency of treatment	The duration of the treatment is nine months in an open group with a frequency of once a week (75 minutes)
Attainment goals	The client has greater insight into his/her own emotions and has learned to better regulate these emotions, as shown by less intense reactions to emotional matters, quicker recovery from intense emotions and a reduced incidence of unacceptable behaviour in response to strong emotions. The client shows more targeted, functional behaviour and less emotion-driven behaviour. The client can now tolerate strong emotions and/or search for distraction when needed

Summary of Dialectical Behaviour Therapy

Dialectical behaviour therapy is a cognitive-behavioural therapy with a broad basis specially developed for people with borderline personality disorders (Linehan, 1996).

The most important characteristic of the theory is recognition that the core disturbance in cases of borderline personality disorder is emotional dysregulation. It is regarded as a consequence of biological disposition, environmental factors and the interaction between the two during the course of an individual's development. The dysregulation is caused by emotional vulnerability and by poorly adapted and inadequate strategies for the regulation of emotions.

Emotional vulnerability has the following characteristics:

1. A very high level of sensitivity to emotional stimuli
2. Strong reactions to emotional stimuli
3. Slow return to the basic emotional level following emotional stimulation

In dialectical behaviour therapy, everything is aimed at teaching clients to regulate their emotions. In a well-functioning family, children receive regular and open confirmation of what they experience. A child's preferences are taken into consideration; parents ask about the opinions and thoughts of the child and take them seriously. The emotions shown by the child are viewed as an important source of information. As a result of adequate and accepting reactions from parents, children are better able to distinguish their own emotions from those of others. However, certain factors can lead to insufficient attention for the child and his or her emotions, which may result in borderline issues.

The behavioural characteristics of borderline clients can be seen as the effects of emotional dysregulation. Impulsive behaviour, particularly harmful behaviour, can be construed as poorly adapted but very effective strategies for the regulation of emotions. In the short term, such behaviours can reduce anxiety, provide distraction and/or mobilise help from the environment. The incapacity to regulate emotional excitement hinders the development of a stable sense of self and the normal expression of emotions, which can quickly give rise to confusion in relationships. Successful relationships are built on a capacity to regulate emotions on your own and a capacity to handle painful stimuli in a functional manner. The capacity to regulate emotions is therefore critical, and its absence leads to behavioural disturbances, mainly in goal-directed and social behaviour.

Dealing with emotions is the capacity to:

1. Suppress inappropriate behaviour associated with strongly negative or positive emotions
2. Undertake intentional action for an external goal that is not mood-dependent
3. Regulate the physiological arousal elicited by the emotions
4. Direct attention to something else when a strong emotion is present

Characteristics of a Personality Disorder According to Linehan

1. Emotional dysregulation
   - extreme emotional sensitivity
   - strong mood fluctuations
   - intense emotional reactions
   - chronic depression
   - problems with anger (restrained or uncontrolled)
2. Interpersonal dysregulation
   - intense and unstable relationships
   - conflictual relationships
   - panic, anxiety and shock or dismay when a relationship ends
   - efforts to avoid abandonment
3. Self-dysfunction
   - chronic emptiness
   - difficulty in asserting own emotions, opinions and decisions in the presence of others
4. Behavioural dysregulation
   - self-damaging behaviour (alcohol, drugs, eating, money, spending money, sex, speeding, etc.)
   - para-suicidal behaviour (self-harm via cutting, pill-taking, etc.)
   - impulsiveness
5. Cognitive dysregulation
   - brief psychotic cognitive disturbances such as depersonalisation, dissociation and delusion, etc.
   - inability to trust

Treatment

The treatment for borderline personality disorder using dialectical behaviour therapy is characterised by the belief that the client has a deeply rooted desire to grow and develop, as well as the belief in an individual's capacity to change.

The term dialectical refers to the view that reality consists of opposing forces (thesis and antithesis). Out of the synthesis of these opposing forces, new opposing forces can emerge. In the therapy, three important polarities are dealt with.

a. The necessity of accepting yourself as you are versus the necessity to change
b. Getting what you need versus losing what you need as your competence increases (e.g. independence versus protection/caring/dependence)
c. Hanging on to your individuality versus acknowledgement of problems and learning new skills to deal with the problems.

Dealing with these polarities means working on the further development of a person's individuality and skills. The treatment is therefore not aimed at maintaining a stable, balanced environment, but at helping the client feel comfortable with change.

For these purposes, the following four modules are used.

- Mindfulness skills, with the objective of learning to be the boss of your mind.
- Emotion regulation skills, with the objective of discovering, understanding and learning to deal with your own emotions in a functional manner.
- Interpersonal effectiveness skills, with the objective of learning to ask for what you need, learning to say no and learning to deal with conflict.
- Distress tolerance skills, with the objective of learning to tolerate and survive crises, but also to accept life as it is now.

The mindfulness module is presented in blocks of two sessions, repeated throughout the course of treatment and alternating with six sessions of the other modules. Once the modules have all been conducted, the cycle is repeated. The idea behind this repetition is that it will help make the knowledge and practice presented more lasting.

8
Mindfulness Module

8.1 Summary of Mindfulness Skills Theory

Mindfulness skills or core mindfulness skillsare central to dialectical behaviour therapy skills training. These skills are learned and then repeated at the beginning of each module. The object of mindfulness skills is learning to be the boss of your own mind. Mindfulness is sometimes referred to as a state of awareness or wholeness (Fig. 8.1).

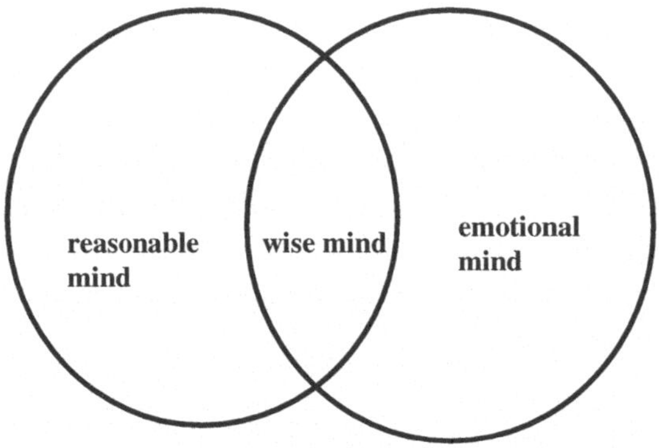

Fig. 8.1 Learning guide 1 (Linehan, 1996)

S. Haeyen, *Art Therapy and Emotion Regulation Problems*,
https://doi.org/10.1007/978-3-319-96773-8_8

There are **three states of mind**:
Reasonable or rational mind: thinking logically, reasoning, concentrating attention, keeping a clear head. To be borne in mind here: the rational mind is important (it is useful; it is easier to think rationally when you feel good, advantages and disadvantages).
Emotional mind: cognitions are 'too hot to touch', it is difficult to think sensibly, objectively, logically, facts are exaggerated or twisted so that they correspond to the current emotional state. The emotional mind is stimulated by (1) illness, (2) lack of sleep, fatigue, (3) drugs, alcohol, (4) hunger, overeating, poor nutrition, (5) stress from one's surroundings (too many demands, claims) and (6) threatening surroundings. To be borne in mind here, the emotional mind is important because it is useful, advantageous; it allows you to compare short-term and long-term consequences, advantages and disadvantages.
Wise mind: the integration of the rational and the emotional mind, the wise mind adds intuitive knowledge to emotional experience and logical analysis. The wise mind is present when a person knows something in a well-balanced, level-headed manner. Everyone has a wise mind; it can be likened to having a heart, or to intuition, but some people have never experienced it, and you cannot continually have a wise mind. You can only learn to use your wise mind with a lot of practice. To be borne in mind here: the wise mind combines knowledge and intuition.

Mindfulness skills are ways of bringing the emotional mind and the rational mind into balance and thus arriving at the wise mind.

There are three *what skills* (observe, describe, participate) and three *how skills* (non-judgementally, one-mindfully, effectively). The purpose of the what skills is to develop an attitude to life characterised by conscious and deliberate participation. Participation without awareness is considered characteristic of impulsive and mood-dependent behaviour, which tends to cause problems.

Observe: Observing and paying attention to events, emotions and behavioural reactions without necessarily trying to stop them even when they are painful, or trying to prolong them when they are pleasant. Learning to let yourself experience a situation purposely, no matter what happens, rather than trying to escape or to put a stop to an emotion.

Describe: Description is a reaction to observation: describing and labelling events and happens and to improve it. This capacity to label (and as a result, to gain distance from emotions as opposed to becoming one with them) is essential for communication and for self-control.

Participate: Participating without focusing on yourself; acting spontaneously. Thoughtful attention means you participate attentively; inattention means you participate inattentively. Participating is ultimately the object of observing and describing.

The *how skills* are about being non-judgemental, about the non-biased perception and observation of behaviour and events. People with borderline issues tend to judge themselves and others in terms that are either overly positive or overly negative. The how skills are not about learning nuances or fine-tuning, but basically involve omitting opinions.

Being non-judgemental: Not forming an opinion about what you observe or describe, or what you participate in. Describing the consequences of what a person does involves observation, but not a moral judgement. This is a difficult point, because people readily tend to judge. When people proffer judgements, do not be disapproving; sometimes, it is important to judge, but most people judge far too often, most often about themselves.

Doing one thing at a time: Learning to concentrate your thoughts on one thing and not allowing yourself to be distracted by thoughts or images from the past, concerns about the future or the presence of negative moods. Learning to control your attention. It is important to give your full attention to what you are doing at that particular time. This applies to both mental and physical activities; however, you can switch from one activity to another.

Acting effectively: Aiming at what works instead of focusing on what is correct or fair. It is the opposite of acting against your own interests. Doing what works means that you must know the object or purpose of what you are doing. It means taking people as they are; something that works in one situation does not always work in another. Acting effectively sometimes means sacrificing principles to achieve a goal. Analysing your own behaviour helps you to understand yourself, your feelings and your behaviour.

8.2 Multidisciplinary Relationships in the Various Aspects of Treatment

Dialectical behaviour therapy Module: Core mindfulness skills	
Being the boss of your own mind, of your behaviour, by working on achieving a balance between the emotional mind and the rational mind (the wise mind) Skills: –what skills: observe, describe, participate –how skills: being non-judgemental, doing one thing at a time, acting effectively	
Skills training	Psycho-education: Learning to take some emotional distance helps you to be less overwhelmed by emotions Analyse your behaviour, seeking a balance
Homework	Assignment: complete the behavioural analysis on conduct that gets in the way of therapy, substance abuse, self-harm, behaviour that obstructs quality of life
Basic group	Unstructured group in which, for example, experiences with emotion-driven behaviour can be discussed
Art therapy	Increasing your sense of perception when viewing expressive works made by yourself and others. Describing rather than judging. Distinguishing between observation and interpretation. Exploring whether the works produced by group members are based on emotions or on rational thinking. Exploring the analogy between your personal works and daily life—for example, by representing the learning guide of the mood circles (rational, emotional and wise mind) in an art work
Music therapy	Watching and observing. Listening to other group members performing and describing what you have heard Participating and making step-by-step plans about how you will participate. Doing one thing at a time. Focusing your attention on performing non-judgementally. Forms of musical performance are diverse. Attention is primarily focused on your interaction with it

Psychomotor therapy	Standing still, observing and describing bodily signals (e.g. basic stance) Observing others and the space around you (becoming aware of place in the space around you) Becoming aware of how exertion affects you (after exerting yourself, you become aware of heat, your heartbeat, your breathing) and psycho-education
Sociotherapy Opening/ closing the daily session, surroundings	Closing the daily session: how would you like to do this and is it a good idea for now, or should you do something different? If you are concerned about being overwhelmed by emotions, take some distance, make a list, enlist help if necessary. Do one thing at a time. Draw up a plan or schedule

8.3 ASSIGNMENT 1: States of Mind/Circles

The illustration is the three states of mind (rational, emotional and wise mind), see the mindfulness model as shown in the two overlapping circles in the introduction. For each part, investigate how that state of mind looks right now for you personally, in form, line and colour.
It may be helpful to consider a difficult situation in your life at present.

OBJECT:

Understanding of and insight into the three states of mind, applied to yourself.
Being the boss of your mind.
Concentrating on one thing at a time, gaining control of your attention.
Practising the what skills and the how skills.

MATERIALS:

Paint or pastels.
Large format paper (70 × 100 cm).
Outline shape for circles and thick black marker to draw the circles.

INDIVIDUALLY in the Group

EXPLANATORY NOTES:

The theory of the three states of mind becomes personal when clients give shape to them in art therapy. This shows which state of mind receives the most attention or is dominant and what issues arise in the three areas. It also shows to what extent a state of mind is integrated for that person. Giving shape to the various aspects is helpful to the process of gaining insight and integrating the states of mind in the person.
Variations to this exercise can be made, for example, by adding text or material from magazines, by having clients develop the three states of mind spatially or by symbolising them in a landscape.
In a later phase, clients can continue to work and develop one aspect, or give shape to the learning goal related to this in a personal work.

EVALUATION:

- What do the states of mind look like in you (observe and describe non-judgementally) and what does this mean?
- Which side do you know well, which side less well?
- What are the advantages and disadvantages of each side? What causes problems, what has advantages and how effective are they?
- What is your learning goal or the point you want to work on?

8.4 ASSIGNMENT 2: Awareness Exercise

The therapist explains:
'A sheet of A2 format paper is taped to the table in front of you. Take a piece of chalk in each hand.
Please sit, relaxed, in your chair, let your arms rest on the paper, with your feet under your knees and pointing straight ahead, your shoulders low. Feel how your chair supports you. If you like, you may close your eyes so you can concentrate better.
Imagine that your flow of thought, which is continuous, comes directly out of your hand, via the chalk, onto the paper. Set your chalk on the paper and let your hands move to the movement of your flow of thought. Keep doing this.
See how this develops for you. Perhaps your thoughts are big, perhaps there are many small thoughts, or so many thoughts that your movements are quick, or perhaps there are few thoughts, your movements are slow ... Observe how your pieces of chalk move around the paper, guided by you. Take time to observe how this is going for you.
Only observe, do not form an opinion, be alert to thoughts that arise in you, don't reject anything, don't cling ...
When a feeling or thought enters your mind, or when you do something, acknowledge it; give the experience words in your thoughts.
Repeat the movement that goes with it. Imprint this in your mind. It is important that you simply do things, and do not form an opinion about what you do. Once you have imprinted this movement in your mind, let it go. Reduce your pressure on the chalk and return your attention to this room ... This is the end of the exercise'.

OBJECT:

Experiencing your own feelings, thoughts, actions.
Focusing attention (on the moment, on your own acts, your own inner movement).
Observing non-judgementally.

MATERIALS:

Pastels, A2 paper, tape.

INDIVIDUALLY in the Group

EXPLANATORY NOTES:

This exercise is an illustration of the mindfulness skills: awareness, focusing attention, observing non-judgementally and consciously letting go of things that occupy you. It is meant as a warming-up exercise, but can also be expanded into an assignment in which clients can develop what they made in the first part into a further, more personal work.

EVALUATION:

- What did this exercise evoke in you? What happened, and how did that feel?
- What kinds of thoughts came into your head, and how did you handle them?
- Did you manage not to be judgemental but merely to observe, notice?
- Were you able to stay with a feeling or thought and then let it go later?
- What skills have you mastered and what skills need some more practice?

8.5 ASSIGNMENT 3: A Theme That Is Important to You in Your Treatment

Decide for yourself what theme is truly important to you at this point in your treatment; what is the focus, or what should be the focus?
Give this shape in an expressive work. You may do this concretely, symbolically, figuratively, or abstractly, but be sure to do it in your own way.

OBJECT:

Becoming aware of the focus of attention of the treatment at this time.
Focusing attention, concentrating on one thing at a time.
Letting go of distraction or avoidance, which steers your attention away from what is important.

MATERIALS:

Free choice.

INDIVIDUALLY in the Group

EXPLANATORY NOTES:

A variation on this could be to make it a feedback assignment in the group, the starting point being that clients make a work for each other (e.g. for the person sitting to their right or left) with the theme of 'Your problem is …'

In the follow-up discussion, it is important to pay attention to whether the work and what is said about it is congruent; does it fit together well, are they in keeping with each other, or do certain striking aspects suggest that it is rationalised or that the expressive work has not been brought to life? If this is the case, it can be linked to the process in the treatment at the time.

EVALUATION:

- For you, what is the most important theme in the treatment right now? Were you able to narrow down your choice?
- How did you represent it?
- How did you use the materials?
- Do others in the group recognise this theme for the person who made the work? (question for the group members)
- Does the theme show itself in the manner of working?

8.6 ASSIGNMENT 4: Hard–Soft Contrasts in Clay

Everyone takes some clay. Warming up with clay (10 minutes); everyone is asked to focus attention on himself or herself and how they personally experience the assignment.

First knead the clay thoroughly and use plenty of energy to make the clay nice and soft. Now, work the clay, but only with your fingertips. Now, work the clay with your entire hand. Feel the difference between pushing hard and using little energy.

Now, starting from the hard–soft contrast, make something out of the clay using the same piece you used for the warming up (30 minutes).

When everyone is finished, first write down on a sheet of paper what everyone observed about himself or herself while working.

OBJECT:

Learning to observe yourself.
Gaining insight.

MATERIALS:

Clay, a base on which to work, clay-working tools.

INDIVIDUALLY in the Group

EXPLANATORY NOTES:

The warming-up exercise can be varied according to the situation.

On the basis of the hard–soft contrast, it may become clear what hard and soft sides the client has (e.g. trust-distrust, needing love-being hurt, judging yourself harshly-being gentle for yourself).

EVALUATION:

- What were your observations of yourself while working the clay?
- Based on your observations, how do you view yourself? (Are your observations reasonably objective or are they highly negative? How realistic is this?)
- In how far does the hard–soft contrast apply to you? Do other group members recognise this? (feedback on observations)

8.7 ASSIGNMENT 5: Contrast in Lines

Put 2 sheets of paper and drawing materials on the table. Sit down, relaxed, focus your attention on yourself and observe how you feel right now.

Choose a piece of chalk in a colour that appeals to you right now. Draw lines based on the movement that fits with how you feel, or that presents itself. Keep doing this for a little while, then use some more energy. You can do this, for example, by going faster or slower, pushing harder or not so hard with the chalk, or by making the movement bigger or smaller (do this for at least 5 minutes).

Now, go to the second sheet and concentrate on the opposite feeling; draw lines or scribble in the way that is appropriate to this. Observe what it is like to do this, and see whether you can step this up (also 5 minutes).

The third step is to combine the two sheets into a single final work. The two sheets can be cut, torn, glued and painted.

OBJECT:

Training what skills and how skills. Self-observation.
Gaining insight into your own opposites and contrasts that can be seen in your emotions, actions and behaviour.
Stimulating integrative skills.

MATERIALS:

Pastels, 2 sheets of white paper 50 × 65 cm, glue, scissors, paint, etc.

INDIVIDUALLY in the Group

EXPLANATORY NOTES:

There may be a contraindication for this exercise if there is too much anxiety, i.e. a client does not know where this will lead him or her; in other words, if a client is too fearful of losing control or is insufficiently prepared to look at his or her own work as a form of expression of their own being.
Combining contrasts by means of an unconscious process.

EVALUATION:

First individual aspects of the contrast are looked at:

- What sort of movement or what kinds of lines did you make and how would you describe them? What are your associations with them, what sort of feeling is appropriate here? (for both sides of the contrast)
- What was the opposite? How would you describe this?

How did you combine the two contrasting sides?

- What do the two sides do with each other? Which side is dominant, or were they in equilibrium?
- Do you recognise in yourself the contrast you have expressed?

8.8 ASSIGNMENT 6: Head and Heart

Make an expressive work on the basis of the theme 'head and heart'. You may do this in whatever way suits you best, as long as the theme is related to yourself. In working it out, show how you experience this theme. For example, think about how much space you want to allot to head and to heart, and about how they are connected.

OBJECT:

Gaining insight into how your own head and heart are connected and related.
Giving artistic expression to and acknowledging personal experience.
Accepting yourself.
Practising the what skills and the how skills.

MATERIALS:

Free choice.

INDIVIDUALLY in the Group

EXPLANATORY NOTES:

In carrying out this assignment, it is important that clients are completely free to connect with it, so that it will have a personal meaning.

EVALUATION:

During the evaluation, a clear distinction must be made between description, observation, emotion and interpretation so that clients practise the mindfulness skills.
Questions focused on gaining insight:
- Which is more familiar to you, your head or your heart; where do you encounter difficulties and how is that shown in the work you have made?
- How are the two parts of your work connected, and what does this tell you?
- Do you recognise how you deal with things, and do group members recognise the images made by other clients?

8.9 ASSIGNMENT 7: Portrait—Blind Drawing

The group members sit down across from each other with a sheet of paper in front of them.

The therapist instructs:
'Take drawing materials and try to draw each other without looking at the paper. Keep the drawing materials in contact with the paper as much as possible. The time for a drawing is short (a few minutes) so that by changing places, each group member can draw all other members once. Use the entire sheet of paper. For the drawing materials, choose from the following options:
- charcoal or black marker (work out using acrylic paint),
- black marker (go over it later with craft glue, and after it dries, work in liquid watercolours) so that black-and-white lines result,
- white oil pastel chalk (work out using liquid watercolours, white lines only become "visible" later)'.

After all group members have been drawn, clients may choose one or two portraits of themselves to work out further.

OBJECT:

Making contact (eye contact) without needing to say anything.
Learning to work non-judgementally.
Observing well and transposing this directly into a movement.
Learning to accept losing some control and learning to play.

MATERIALS:

White A4 paper.
Marker, transparent craft glue, liquid watercolours, charcoal, acrylic paints.

IN PAIRS/INDIVIDUALLY

EXPLANATORY NOTES:

In this assignment, funny or strange drawings may surprise you; in fact, they cannot fail to. If the portrait is a good resemblance, someone probably cheated; this is a good reason not to mind if your portrait does not look like you or your model, and it makes it easier to take part non-judgementally. In fact, it is great fun. Because you must work quickly and may not look at what you draw, this assignment has a lower threshold. It can be even further enhanced by drawing with your left hand (if you are right-handed) or vice versa.
If you think that people will try to sneak a look anyway, you can put a thin plastic sheet or cloth over the drawing area, so that people can work under it.

EVALUATION:

- What do you think of the drawing?
- Is there some resemblance? (an odd-looking drawing can still show something of the person who was the model)
- How did you like drawing and not being able to see what you drew, meaning that you had less control?
- How did it look when you worked it out?

8.10 ASSIGNMENT 8: Drawing by Feeling

Put some paint on a flat surface (glass or smooth wood) and roll it out with a paint roller. Put a sheet of paper over it. Using your finger(s) or nail(s), make an imaginary drawing on the paper. Feel the paper and try to discover the difference between soft and hard, working with your flat hand and/or with sharp nails. Take the paper off the panel or slate and look at the result. This process can be repeated several times to experiment with it. Then one of the paint drawings can be selected to work out in more detail.

OBJECT:

Becoming aware of the touch organs, stimulating the senses.
Allowing yourself to experiment.

MATERIALS:

Smooth surface on which to roll out the paint, block print paints (oily, does not dry quickly), paint rollers, cords or other materials to experiment with.

INDIVIDUALLY in the Group

EXPLANATORY NOTES:

This assignment can also be done in pairs, which may encourage experimentation.

EVALUATION:

- What was it like to feel your way in painting?
- Was your touch hard or gentle, did you use your flat hand, fingertips or nails?
- What did you like about it, what did you not like?
- Did you try out different ways? Did you discover anything?

8.11 ASSIGNMENT 9: Chalk Scribbles

The steps in this assignment are offered by the therapist one at a time.

'Put four sheets of A4 paper in front of you. From the box with oil pastels, choose four colours that appeal to you. Take them out and place them with your paper'.

'Now take one colour and scribble something on the first sheet. Take the second colour and scribble on the second sheet. Do the same with the following sheets: a third colour for the third sheet and a fourth colour for the fourth sheet'.

'Go back to the first sheet and finish the picture using the other colours. Go on to the second sheet and finish this picture, and do the same with the third and the fourth sheets'.

'Think up a word or title for the first picture and write this down. Do the same for the second, third and fourth pictures'.

'Now make a sentence or a short story from the words (1–4). It does not need to be imaginative'.

OBJECT:

Increasing spontaneity.
Submitting to a process without deciding everything yourself or rationalising.
Discovering emotional content.
Increasing insight into your own pattern, how you assign meaning.

MATERIALS:

Oil pastels, per person 4 sheets of A4 paper.

INDIVIDUALLY in the Group

EXPLANATORY NOTES:

The therapist uses a directive approach for carrying out this assignment step by step while keeping things moving. This means that the therapist must keep a close eye on the time and must give clear instructions.
The basic idea is not to spend time thinking about the assignment or controlling or influencing the final result. It is important to allow yourself to be led and to leave room for surprises and spontaneity. Sometimes, this assignment proves to be fun: then it is simply about what you are doing, and no personal themes present themselves. However, it can also be confrontational and revealing, even though this may not have been the client's intention.

EVALUATION:

- What was it like to do this assignment?
- Could you please show the pictures in order and tell us your sentence or story?
- Do you recognise certain themes that come forward here? Was this something you focused on while working, or did you not see a relationship until later?
- If you did not recognise a personal theme, is this an outcome you can accept?

8.12 ASSIGNMENT 10: Individual Silhouette

Hang a large sheet of paper on the wall. One person stands in front of it in a self-chosen posture. Let this person choose who will draw his or her silhouette. The silhouette of the upper body is drawn in pencil by the person selected. Then the silhouette is developed and worked out by the person who was the model for it. Make the line black using a marker; you could also go over it again with glue to make a shiny transparent layer over the black. Go on to experiment with liquid watercolours to fill out the silhouette.

OBJECT:

Self-observation: practising what skills and how skills.
Participation: opening yourself to experimentation.

MATERIALS:

Large sheet of paper (70 × 100 cm) per person. Pencil, marker, transparent paper glue, liquid watercolours, paintbrush, sponge, water, etc.

INDIVIDUALLY in the Group

EXPLANATORY NOTES:

Letting the person being silhouetted choose the one who will do this is important because the latter comes quite close and this creates tension. The person being silhouetted is also the centre of attention, because the other group members are there and observe. Because the model makes this choice, he or she retains autonomy but is also asked to surrender to the situation.

If you decide to cover the line with glue, consider how long it will take to dry so that you can continue working.

EVALUATION:

- Describe what you observed in yourself while your silhouette was being drawn.
- Was it exciting, suspenseful, and how did you react to this? What did the others discern about you? (question for the group members)
- Were you able to allow yourself this experience, without stopping the experience or the emotion and without wanting to make it last longer either?
- What do you look like on the picture, how did you develop it further? Describe your work.

8.13 ASSIGNMENT 11: Four Exercises on Observing

1. Sit down in a way that is comfortable. Breathe in and out deeply three times. Observe in yourself how you feel inside at this time. And how do you feel in relation to your surroundings?

This is followed by a very brief round about how each group member feels, making a distinction into inner feelings and feelings in relation to the surroundings. This can also be done by asking group members to very quickly (in a few minutes) draw something to represent the experience or to describe it in a single word.

2. Drawing on someone's back: exercise in pairs. Number one takes chalk and paper, number two sits behind number one and draws something on number one's back, using his or her finger or the end of a paintbrush or pencil. Number one tries to draw on the paper what he or she feels is being drawn on his or her back. Then change places.

This is followed by a brief round about how this went, and which role (leading or following) they enjoyed most. People often tend to try to second-guess what the other one means, and to fill in what they think the drawing will show. This happens in ordinary conversations as well: a tendency to say what you think the other person will say, what he or she means, before that person has finished speaking.

3. Leading/following: One person in the group is the leader. The others follow. The leader has a linear drawing (or picture) in front of him or her and describes it for the others, who cannot see the drawing (as if, during a telephone

conversation, you want to show the person you are talking to exactly what the picture or drawing, which you have in front of you, looks like). The group members try to draw the drawing on the basis of the description.

Brief round in which the results are viewed.

4. Leading/following: One person is the leader. Instead of a drawing, he or she thinks about his or her living room and describes to the others what it looks like. The others draw the living room according to what this person says. There is a brief follow-up discussion.

This exercise is sometimes even more difficult than number 3 because you know your own living room so well: how can you tell others about it as objectively as possible?

OBJECT:

Practising the what skills and the how skills; observe, describe, participate non-judgementally, do one thing at a time.
Learning to lead and to follow.

MATERIALS:

A3 paper, crayon, a linear drawing for exercise 3.

INDIVIDUALLY/IN PAIRS/IN THE GROUP

EXPLANATORY NOTES:

Clients may experience having a drawing made on their back as exciting or provocative. Some ways of dealing with this: draw with the end of the paintbrush, agree that one of you can say stop, make a drawing on a person's hand instead of their back.

Observing, describing and being clear towards others are often more difficult than it seems. In the drawings, it can immediately be seen what goes wrong, and how much goes wrong, in reproducing a picture described in words. From here is it easy to make the link to other situations in which your own information may come across incorrectly or in which you interpret information incorrectly by not observing properly.

EVALUATION:

Following each exercise, experiences are shared. After the series of exercises, the experience can be linked, for example, to observing in conversations and how clearly you express what you want to say.

8.14 ASSIGNMENT 12: Clay Sphere

Make two large, smooth half-spheres of the same size from clay, using the ring technique. Fix the two halves of the sphere together by scraping and using clay silt so that a hollow clay sphere results. Now, make an opening in the sphere where you let something come out that is also made of clay. This can be just about anything. Follow whatever occurs to you.

OBJECT:

Working on the basis of a structure.
Drawing from your imagination.
Gaining insight into your thoughts or perceptions.
Gaining self-insight.

MATERIALS:

Clay (coarse/fine chamotte), base, spatulas, sculpting tools, battens.

INDIVIDUALLY in the Group

EXPLANATORY NOTES:

The sphere construction requires working with concentration on the basis of a structure: making clay rings, building the sphere shape, attaching the rings tightly, making the shape sturdy. Sometimes it is difficult to make the two halves of equal size so as to wind up with a round shape.

The second part of this exercise requires imagination, allowing yourself to follow whatever comes into your head.

EVALUATION:

- What was it like to make the clay sphere?
- Did you encounter any difficulties?
- What comes out of your sphere? What made you think of that?
- What feeling does this put across?
- What does it say about you? Do you recognise it?

8.15 ASSIGNMENT 13: Basic Forms

Choose from the following basic forms: cross, circle, square, spiral or triangle. Each of these forms may call to mind entirely different things. As a stimulus, the group can take a brief look at each of the forms.

Make a painting based on the form you chose, and see what it invites you to do. Work so that the entire sheet is covered with paint.

OBJECT:

- Gaining insight into your own perception and how you assign meaning.
- Investigating your own behaviour in the medium.
- Observing basic forms and what they call to mind, what they invite you to do.

MATERIALS:

Acrylic paints, several paintbrushes and paper.

INDIVIDUALLY in the Group

EXPLANATORY NOTES:

Every basic shape is a Gestalt with a certain meaning or emotional meaning. In the follow-up discussion, the therapist can perhaps say something about the information in the literature (*Riedel, I., Formen, Tiefenpsychologische Deutung von Kreis, Kreuz, Dreieck, Quadrat, Spirale und Mandala, 2002, Kreuz Verlag GmbH & Co. KG Stuttgart, Zürich*).

The circle stands for infinity, belonging, security, being enclosed, for the centre or core and surroundings. The square stands for boundaries, being enclosed, separated or defined, and angles. The spiral stands for symbols of development, life, looking from the present to the future, a free form, dynamic. The cross stands for a variety of force fields (north-south, east-west and over-under, right-left), opposites, tensions and bringing them together, orientation on opposing feelings or forces. The triangle stands for linked tensions, balance and variable force fields.

EVALUATION:

- How did you arrive at your choice of a shape?
- Describe what you did with it.
- Do you recognise the possible meaning of the basic shape? (*information from the book*)
- What is your own meaning or interpretation of it in the work you made?
- What is the link to your own themes/issues?

8.16 ASSIGNMENT 14: Imagination—The Seed

The therapist asks briefly about previous experiences with guided imagery. If necessary, the therapist explains how the assignment will take place.

The participants are asked to sit up straight, feet on the floor, arms resting on their legs. Before the guided imagery, there is a relaxation exercise.

The therapist instructs:
'Imagine that you are a tiny seed, that you are underground, in the earth ... it's dark and the soil may feel a bit damp ...Slowly, you feel that something is changing, you are changing and starting to grow ... you fight your way up, towards the air and the light ... when you first come above the ground, you feel the warmth of the sunlight ... you go on growing and you produce leaves ... what do they look like, are they large or small, are they prickly or smooth, what colour are they? You go on growing and perhaps you even produce flowers or fruits; what do they look like? You grow as big as you imagine you are ... Take a good look at yourself; what do you look like? Imprint this picture in your mind ... Now look around you, look at your surroundings ... what does it look like around you? Are there other plants too? And what does the landscape look like? Is it warm or cold, is it dry or damp? Do you feel the wind, or is there no wind? Imprint this picture in your mind too ... Then look again at yourself and hold onto this picture ... Now gradually return your attention to this room and this time; when you are here, open your eyes ...'

'Now use the materials to make the images that you saw'.

OBJECT:

Gaining insight into your own perception via a more or less subconscious process.

MATERIALS:

Pastels, acrylic paints and paper

INDIVIDUALLY in the Group

EXPLANATORY NOTES:

Some clients find it difficult or frightening to think about their own body, about relaxing. Sometimes images become blocked. The theme 'under the ground' may lead to an oppressive association, but once the plant begins to grow, this generally disappears.

EVALUATION:

- What was it like to do this exercise? Were you able to relax, did you see images, what happened with you during the guided imagery?
- What sort of picture did you see? Describe it. What in the picture was important for you?
- What can we see in the work you made (line, forms, colours, atmosphere, substance)?
- What does the work tell you? Does the person who made it recognise this content? And do others?

8.17 ASSIGNMENT 15: Draw the Core Quadrant

Everyone makes their own core quadrant (Daniel Ofman) and fills in their personal quality and other words fitting the quadrant.

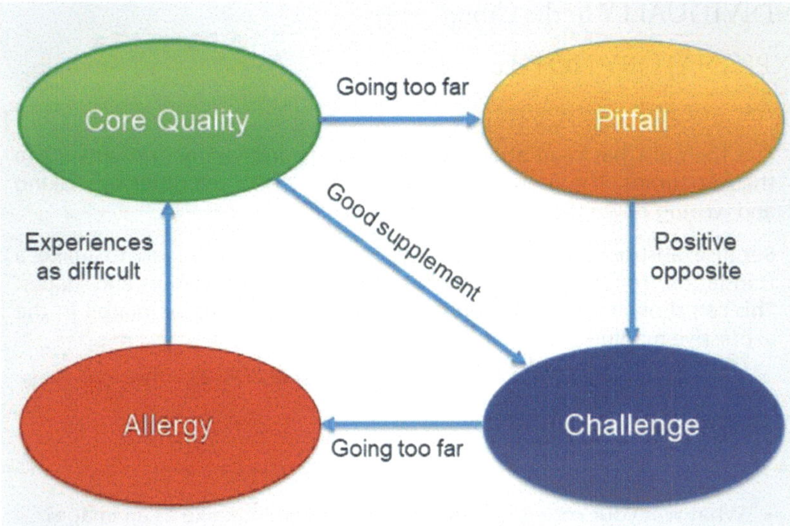

Core quadrant (Van Vliet, 2012).

Then everyone makes four abstract paintings on A4 paper to go with the four sides of the quadrant. They are pasted on a large sheet of paper in the way they are ordered in the core quadrant, producing an expressive quadrant. The challenge may coincide with or be appropriate to one of the client's treatment goals.

OBJECT:

Gaining insight into your own quality, pitfall, allergy and challenge. Investigating and determining the direction of your personal development.

MATERIALS:

Painting materials, 4 sheets of A4 paper and 1 large sheet (70 × 100 cm) per person.

INDIVIDUALLY in the Group

EXPLANATORY NOTES:

The therapist has read about core quadrants and can help clients make their quadrant. The group members can also help each other by making and writing down the core quadrants in pairs.

Because abstract design is required, clients are encouraged to make a translation from the core quadrant to the use of lines, colours and shapes. This can show where a challenge or treatment goal can be placed in the expressive medium, where it becomes clear.

EVALUATION:

- What was your core quadrant and what did it look like as an image?
- What does this mean for the further course of art therapy? Can you link an expressive objective to this?

8.18 ASSIGNMENT 16: Imagination—The Conveyor Belt

Paper and drawing materials are on the table.
We start with an imagination exercise, followed by the assignment.

The therapist instructs:
'Would you all please sit relaxed in your chair, put your arms on the arm rests, with your feet under your knees and pointing straight ahead, your shoulders low. Feel how your chair supports you. If you like, you may close your eyes so as to concentrate better'.

'Imagine that your flow of thought, a continuous stream, has the form of a conveyor belt. How does it work for you? There may be a few large packages on it, or many smaller ones; there may be so much on it that the packages are almost falling off the belt, or perhaps a package only comes by every now and then. Take your time to observe how this looks for you right now. Don't think that there should be more packages or fewer packages, or that they need to be red or blue. Just observe the picture you see non-judgmentally'.

'Now I want you all to pick up a package from the belt in your mind and to take a good look at it from all sides. It is important that you only look, and do not form an opinion about the package. Feel whether it is light or heavy. Open the package and see what is inside it. Once you have imprinted this in your mind, close the package, put it back on the conveyor belt and let go of it. The belt will take the package with it'.

'Let's leave the conveyor belt and come back to the room here. This is the end of the exercise.

'Now, based on this exercise, make a drawing of the package, of its content or of the conveyor belt. You will have plenty of time for this'.

OBJECT:

Awareness
Directing attention
Observing non-judgementally
Letting go of things that occupy your mind.

MATERIALS:

Paper in various formats, several drawing materials.

INDIVIDUALLY in the Group

EXPLANATORY NOTES:

The content of the package may be surprising, and it may make the person doing the exercise aware of something that may be confronting. It is interesting to see what the person then does with it: is it used in the expressive work, or is it kept separate (is it acknowledged or disclaimed?)
It is also striking how differently the conveyor belt may be organised for each person.
People can have very different perceptions of what it is like to put the package back on the conveyor belt and let go of it.

EVALUATION:

- How did the exercise go for you?
- What did your conveyor belt look like? Were there many packages, or few, and were they orderly, or all jumbled together?
- How did it feel to remove one package?
- What did that package look like, and what was in it? Did you make this? How did you imagine it?
- How did it feel to put the package back? Did you want to?
- Looking back, what do you think? What is your conclusion?

8.19 ASSIGNMENT 17: Scribble Drawing

Put a sheet of paper (50 × 65 cm) on the table in front of you and choose one of the coloured pastels that appeals to you. Don't think about it too much, choose intuitively.

Use this colour to draw lines on the sheet of paper. It is not supposed to represent anything in particular. Try out movements to see what you like—round, big, angular or small, using little pressure or lots of pressure. Continue making this movement for 5 or 10 minutes.

Then put the pastel down and brush with your fingers (perhaps with your whole hand) over the pastel lines. Take 5 minutes to do this.

Then choose a second colour and continue working on the drawing.
While you are drawing, let a word occur to you. In the remaining time, develop the expressive work and let the word show up in your drawing.

OBJECT:

Observing your own acts, your inner movement and/or perception.
Doing one thing at a time, gaining control of your attention.

MATERIALS:

Pastel, sheet op paper (50 × 65 cm).

INDIVIDUALLY in the Group

EXPLANATORY NOTES:

It is important that clients work in silence so that everyone can concentrate and be drawn into the making of their work.

EVALUATION:

- What did you observe in yourself while working?
- Could you allow yourself to experience this, without stopping the experience or emotion but without wanting to make it last longer either?
- What did you observe when you brushed the picture with your fingers or hands; did that give you a different feeling?
- What word occurred to you?
- Describe your work as it now looks. What strikes you about it?

8.20 ASSIGNMENT 18: Series of Three Paintings

Take paint in two colours plus black and white paint on a palette.
Take 3 sheets of A3 paper per person.

Take the first sheet of paper and cover it with the paint in a way that represents nothing in particular, in such a way that the sheet of paper is covered completely and none of the paper is visible.
When you have finished the first sheet, take the second sheet. The assignment is the same, but now you may choose to change something, to work it out differently. The colours are still the same; you may not pick a different colour. When the second sheet is finished, take the third sheet (same assignment). You may not alter the paintings you have completed.

OBJECT:

Observing your own reactions and choices during the work process.
Participating.
Describing.

MATERIALS:

Acrylic paint, 3 sheets of A3 paper per person.

INDIVIDUALLY in the Group

EXPLANATORY NOTES:

It is important that the three paintings are made as a series, one by one, without going back or working ahead.

This assignment can also be done in pairs (non-verbally).

By painting the sheet of paper completely, the maker becomes more closely involved with the materials and with the process of painting.

EVALUATION:

- Describe your own series, particularly the process that took place while you painted.
- How did you go from the first work to the second, and to the third; what choices did you make; and what reasons did you have for them?
- What behaviour or choice pattern can be recognised in this process?
- Do you recognise this pattern from other situations?

8.21 ASSIGNMENT 19: Florence Cane* Technique

Hang a large sheet of paper on the wall, or stick it to the table with tape. Take a charcoal crayon in each hand. Close your eyes and concentrate on the crayon and the paper. Pay attention to your posture and make sure your stance is relaxed. Start moving both hands on the paper at the same time and move them continually. The therapist will tell you when to stop. Everyone works like this for 5–10 minutes. Follow your hands and whatever comes into your head.

When the time is up, group members look at and discuss each other's work, how it arose, and what it felt like to do this. After this, everyone continues working on the scribble drawing. You are free in the further development of this drawing, which means, for example, that you can also paint over lines.

OBJECT:

Participating (acting spontaneously).
Observing.

MATERIALS:

Large sheet of paper, 70 × 90 cm.
Charcoal.
Paint or chalk.

INDIVIDUALLY in the Group

EXPLANATORY NOTES:

The drawings can also be worked out in pairs.

* Florence Cane was a drawing teacher at a school in New York. She developed a number of relaxation and drawing exercises with the object of reducing fear of failure, encouraging movement in her students and helping them to be in touch with their own creativity (1983).

EVALUATION:

- What was the first part of this assignment like, when you were not allowed to look, working with both hands at the same time and allowing yourself to be led by what your hands wanted to do by themselves, naturally?
- In the second part, you could decide for yourself. What did you decide to do with the original drawing? Say something about how this went.
- Describe the end result non-judgementally.

8.22 ASSIGNMENT 20: Watercolour Picture

Stick the watercolour paper down with tape on all edges so that later, when the tape is removed, the paper will have a white frame.

Using a sponge and some water, make the entire paper quite moist so that the paint can flow over the paper. Using watercolours and a broad, flat and soft paintbrush, make a picture showing a background of air, land and perhaps water or a sea in a way that it looks the most pleasing to you. Cover the entire sheet of paper. Too much paint can be removed with water or a cloth. Make horizontal strokes with the paintbrush and observe attentively how the paint and the colour flow on the sheet of paper. Pay attention to the moment. (25 mins.)

When the background is finished, the next step is to add something to the background using a finer brush. This can be a detail or more than that. The point is that you follow what is in your mind, that you look to see what the painting needs, in your opinion. Try not to let yourself be led by what you think is 'proper' or ought to be done.

OBJECT:

Learning to surrender to the process without wanting to steer or control it.
Focusing attention, concentrating on one thing at a time.
Discovering the content of your feelings.
Acknowledging your own wishes and needs.

MATERIALS:

Watercolour paper (A2 or A3), watercolour paint, water, sponges, watercolour brushes (both large flat brushes and finer ones), towels/tissues and tape.

INDIVIDUALLY in the Group

EXPLANATORY NOTES:

It is important to explain a bit about watercolour technique so that group members are encouraged to experiment a bit more.

EVALUATION:

- What was it like working with watercolours?
- What was it like to work with such fluid materials? How did you handle them?
- What sort of landscape did you paint?
- What did you add to it?
- Were you able to hold on to what you wanted to do, to your ideas, and not to start doing what you thought you should do, or ought to do?
- What want is shown in the painting (if any)? What do you find striking?

8.23 ASSIGNMENT 21: Painting Experiment

Take a large sheet of paper and fold it so that it has six areas. In each of the areas, try out a different manner of painting. Do this without brushes, but use different materials such as tissues, sponges, washing-up brushes, palette knives and so on. Then take a second sheet of paper and choose one manner of painting that you found to be the most surprising or the most pleasant. Make a larger painting in that manner.

OBJECT:

Allowing yourself to experiment and discover.
Becoming aware of where your preference lies.

MATERIALS:

Various colours of paint, paper 50 × 65 cm, 2 sheets per person, sponge, cloth, washing-up brush, palette knives, sand, water, etc.

INDIVIDUALLY in the Group

EXPLANATORY NOTES:

This assignment encourages clients to investigate different manners of painting. The paint becomes a field of discovery, and not just a means of producing a picture. This allows clients to delve more deeply into the possibilities offered by the materials.

EVALUATION:

- What manners of painting did you discover?
- Which ones appealed to you, and which ones were less appealing?
- Why did a particular manner of working appeal to you?
- How did you continue working in this manner on the second sheet of paper?

8.24 ASSIGNMENT 22: Tearing

Everyone has a sheet of paper. We take 5–10 minutes to tear the paper, in silence and with purposeful attention. Observe what you see, feel, do, think, hear or smell. The therapist will tell you when the time is up.

Experiences in relation to what you have observed will be exchanged in a brief round. After that, group members will make a work in which the bits of torn paper are the starting point. Inspiration can also come from the experience of the first exercise (tearing). More materials may be used for this part.

OBJECT:

Focusing attention.
Consciously observing.
Investigating your own shaping process.

MATERIALS:

Paper, per person at least 1 sheet of paper (50 × 65 cm), for example sketch paper; free choice of additional materials.

INDIVIDUALLY in the Group

EXPLANATORY NOTES:

This exercise combines well with a scribble task in which lines are drawn and then the paper is torn.

Using coloured paper (coloured on one side or both) is another option.

EVALUATION:

- A group round after the first exercise: What did you observe using your senses? Describe this.
- Did you recognise certain characteristic behaviour in yourself, or certain thoughts?
- After making the works, what did you do with the strips, snippets and other bits of paper to make an art work?
- What inspired you?

References

Cane, F. (1983). *The artist in each of us*. New York: Pantheon.

Linehan, M. M. (1996). *Borderline persoonlijkheidsstoornisstoornis. Handleiding voor training en therapie* [Skills training manual for treating borderline personality disorder]. Lisse, The Netherlands: Swets & Zeitlinger.

Van Vliet, V. (2012). *Daniel Ofman*. Retrieved May 23, 2018 from ToolsHero: https://www.toolshero.com/toolsheroes/daniel-ofman/.

9

Emotion Regulation Module

9.1 Summary of Emotion Regulation Skills Theory

From the point of view of dialectical behaviour therapy, problems with regulating painful emotions are key to the behavioural problems of people with borderline disorders. Dysfunctional behaviours such as self-harm, suicidal conduct or substance abuse are often behavioural solutions for unbearably painful emotions.

People frequently tell themselves that they are not allowed to feel what they feel. This is a solution often related to an emotionally debilitating background: one in which they must laugh when they are unhappy, be kind and cooperative when they are angry, admit they are guilty when they do not feel guilty.

Emotions

There are eight primary emotions (anger, sadness, happiness, surprise, fear, disgust, guilt/shame, expectation/interest).

Emotions are specific reaction patterns to events; emotions are complex and are composed of numerous elements. Emotions come and go, and frequently last only a few seconds to minutes. Emotions maintain

S. Haeyen, *Art Therapy and Emotion Regulation Problems*,
https://doi.org/10.1007/978-3-319-96773-8_9

themselves, continually restart themselves. If emotions are more lasting, we refer to this as a mood.

Emotions have a communicative function towards yourself and others: emotions influence and control the behaviour of others; they validate a person's own observations and interpretations of events.

Emotion Regulation means:

Observing and describing emotions

The first step in emotion regulation is learning to recognise and name emotions as they arise. But emotions are complex. It is helpful to observe and describe the following aspects: event, interpretation, sensations, behaviours, after-effects of the emotion.

Emotion regulation demands the non-judgemental observation and description of your own emotional reactions.

Recognising primary emotions

It is thought that much emotional unease arises from secondary reactions (intense shame, anger, fear) to primary emotions. The primary emotions are often appropriate to the context in which they arise. But if they are not allowed to be felt, secondary reactions emerge in which there is much self-punishment, resulting in very painful emotions.

Such secondary reactions can be lessened by exposure to the primary reaction, learning to experience and to tolerate it, in a non-judgemental atmosphere. Once they have been activated, sadness and anger cannot be ignored; they demand a place. Secondary emotions cause all kinds of problems.

Increasing positive emotions

Dialectical behaviour therapy assumes that people feel bad because they have a good reason for it. It is therefore of great importance to augment the number of positive events and devote attention to pleasant experiences when they occur. Clients are encouraged to do positive things, to devote attention to relationships and to shun avoidance.

Tolerating negative emotions without showing impulsive behaviour, which only makes matters worse, is an important way in which to regulate the intensity and duration of negative emotions.

Lessening vulnerability to negative emotions

Emotional reactions are reinforced under the influence of physical stress or stress arising from your surroundings. This is why it is important to lessen your own vulnerability—for instance, by making sure you get enough sleep and eat well—so that you have good resistance to negative emotions. By building up control, you also build up a feeling of trust and competence. This makes you more resistant to negative emotions.

Letting go of emotional suffering: Paying attention to your emotion of the moment

Painful emotions are part of being human. It is often difficult to shake them off. The trick is to find new ways to deal with negative emotions so that they cause less suffering. This can be achieved by accepting them. Acceptance of painful emotions turns off the suffering, leaving only the pain. If you fight emotions, it invariably ensures that they persist.

Acting opposite to the emotion of the moment

Effective therapies for depression, anxiety and dealing with anger all have one characteristic in common: turning emotions into behaviour. In depressions, the behaviour is activated; in anxieties, people are exposed to what makes them anxious, causing the fear or anxiety to fade and end. For anger, people learn to recognise the reason for their anger and simply exit the situation.

Examples of doing the opposite

Fear: do what it is you are afraid of instead of avoiding it. Guilt or shame: don't avoid the emotion, experience it and if necessary, make excuses. Sadness or depression: be active, do not avoid the emotion by remaining passive. Anger: avoid the person you are angry with rather than attacking him or her.

In Brief

By learning to observe emotions, people learn to distance themselves from their emotions, not to become one with them, but nevertheless to form an entity, a whole, with their emotions. In order to control emotions, people must be able to distance themselves so that they can think things over and make use of coping strategies.

9.2 Multidisciplinary Relationships in the Various Aspects of Treatment

Dialectical Behaviour Therapy
Module: Emotion Regulation Skills

Dysfunctional behaviours such as self-harm or substance abuse are often behavioural solution for unbearably painful emotions.

Skills:
- recognising, naming and understanding emotions as a communicative function towards yourself and others
- lessening emotional vulnerability, increasing positive events

Skills training	Psycho-education: necessity of setting limits, tolerating the accompanying tension
Homework	Behavioural analysis in setting limits, observing emotions Completing the behaviour analysis form, discussion of myths about emotions
Basic group	Unstructured group in which participants can talk, for example, about emotions during and after a boundary has been crossed
Art therapy	Recognising and expressively showing emotions in art work but at the same time structuring the emotions by transforming them into understandable and communicative representations. Experiencing individuality, symbolising emotions, giving shape to your self-image (human images or abstract images) or polarities in your character, visualisation, imagination. Use of materials: What is right for me, what is not? Group exercise in giving one another positive feedback on the basis of figures or images (which are then worked out individually)
Music therapy	Exercises for recognising, expressing and meting out emotions Receptive: listening to CDs of other clients Active: various forms. For example, giving emotions musical form. Singing on the basis of various emotions and with attention to expression. Making music together, with emphasis on timing and dealing with structure
Psychomotor therapy	Exercises aimed at control, exploring, observing, feeling emotions in your own body (e.g. starting from the basic emotions), communicating emotions to the other in posture, facial expression and words, ways of moving to reduce vulnerability (e.g. experiencing what forms of movement are suited to you in what situations)

Sociotherapy Opening/closing the daily session, surroundings	At the end of the day, reflecting on how the day went. What moved you, how will you start your evening. Ensure stability by caring for yourself properly: eat healthily, relax with a form of activity, but be sure to have a nice cup of tea now and then

9.3 ASSIGNMENT 1: Emotional Diary

In a diary of emotions, circles are filled in once a day with colours that stand for different emotions. For this purpose, make a book of a number of pages with one large circle on each page. The book is meant to last as long as you want to keep filling it in—as long as the module lasts, for example. Mark the date on each page.

Homework: Every day you fill in a circle. Make a legend showing the meaning you give to colours symbolising one of the basic emotions: sad, afraid, angry, happy.

We assume that each of the emotions is present, to varying degrees, every day.

OBJECT:

Taking a closer look at emotions by observing and learning to recognise, explore and acknowledge feelings and emotions.

MATERIALS:

Paper (A4 or smaller), stapler for books, compass, coloured pencils or pigment sticks.

INDIVIDUALLY

EXPLANATORY NOTES:

Optionally, the circles from a certain period can be used to conclude the therapy; clients can make a summarising work, for example.

EVALUATION:

- When you review a period in your emotional diary, what do you find particularly striking?
- Do certain emotions have a very strong presence, or do certain emotions occur less frequently?
- Can you recognise a pattern?

9.4 ASSIGNMENT 2: You and a Significant Other

Make a human figure out of clay to represent yourself (20 min.). It doesn't have to look just like you. Decide whether you want the figure to be seated, standing or lying down and what expression it should have.

Make a second clay figure representing a significant other (20 min.).

Place the two figures in a way that represents their relationship.

OBJECT:

Obtaining insight into your own self-image in an important relationship.

MATERIALS:

Clay, base to work on, clay-working tools.

INDIVIDUALLY in the Group

EXPLANATORY NOTES:

In part, this assignment shows how the client sees, or would like to see, the relationship with a significant other. The picture may be a realistic or an ideal one.
Sometimes things happen when the clay is shaped that were not intended but that may reveal something unexpected.

EVALUATION:

- How did you represent yourself?
- Who is your significant other?
- Is there some difference or similarity between the two figures?
- How did you position the two figures and what does this say about their relationship?
- Did you make an idealised image or a realistic one?

9.5 ASSIGNMENT 3: Landscape Fantasy

1. Sit down, relax and try to imagine a landscape. (Is it panoramic or secluded, cold or warm, rocky or grassy, damp or dry ...). Write down this information in keywords.
2. Imagine a dwelling or shelter in this landscape. (House, cave, burrow, tree house, etc.)
3. Now, a person appears in the landscape. (What does the person look like: tall, short, young, old, etc.)

4. And now a problem has arisen in this picture; what do you suppose that is?
5. When you have answered all the questions, draw or paint the image in your mind.

OBJECT:

Participating; letting yourself be drawn into a fantasy tale in which you may encounter themes of your own.
Acquiring insight into what is taking place right now in your experiential world.

MATERIALS:

Paints, chalk, paper.

INDIVIDUALLY in the Group

EXPLANATORY NOTES:

The story in the landscape fantasy can also be worked out in comic strip form. It is important to stay close to the fantasy.
Leave clients plenty of freedom to go along with their fantasy.
This assignment can be given as a follow-up to the emotion island, part of which can be used in more detail here.

EVALUATION:

- Share with the group the landscape, the shelter, the protagonist and the problem of your fantasy.
- What sort of relationship has arisen between you and what you created in your surroundings?
- Is the problem familiar to you?

9.6 ASSIGNMENT 4: Emotion in Clay and Other Materials

Choose a strong emotion that you recently had to deal with. Make a clay figure, taking this emotion as the starting point. Combine your work in clay with another material (here the therapist presents a wide range of options, or they may be displayed on the table).

OBJECT:

Giving expression to a strong emotion.
Learning not to lose yourself in this, but to be very clear.
Making strong emotions observable, concrete and open to discussion, showing what is going on and how you deal with it.

MATERIALS:

Clay, clay-working tools.
Other materials to combine with the clay, such as wire, beads, feathers, pebbles, fabrics, bits of glass, wool, paper, newspaper or mosaic tiles.

INDIVIDUALLY in the Group

EXPLANATORY NOTES:

If clients have not previously worked with clay, you might want to start with a brief explanation or a collective warming-up.

EVALUATION:

- Give your work a title and write it down.
  First the group members have their say about the work created, and afterwards the person who made it.
- Ask the group members what associations they have on seeing the work, and what might be a suitable title or name for it.
- After this, the person who made it says his or her own title, explains a bit about the work and responds to the names given to it by the others.

9.7 ASSIGNMENT 5: Powerful—Powerless

Part 1:
Think of a time when you felt very powerful … now make a drawing of it. After this, think of a time when you felt very powerless … and make a drawing of it. For both drawings, you have a total of around 30–40 minutes.

Part 2:
(The second part is not explained until part 1 has been completed.)
Now, write a small piece based on these two works by completing the following lines in your own words. Together, they will form a poem:

1. Right now I would most like to …
2. (where/somewhere)
3. so that everyone (no-one) sees that …
4. so that everyone (no-one) hears that …
5. so that everyone (no-one) knows that …
6. (Join together what you wrote in point 1 and the place you named in point 2 to make a concluding sentence.)

OBJECT:

Expressing emotions of various natures.
Gaining insight into your own experiences and feelings.
Showing who you are in the group by the way you give form to personal experiences, and letting the group share in these experiences and feelings.

MATERIALS:

Drawing and painting materials or whatever you prefer.

INDIVIDUALLY in the Group

EXPLANATORY NOTES:

It may be important to offer some help with writing the verse.

It is possible that in the follow-up discussion, someone does not want to say too much about the situations, but is willing to read out the verse.

EVALUATION:

- What did you make for the first situation?
- Can you read out the poem you made for it?
- What did you make for the second situation?
- Is there a relationship between the powerful and the powerless situation?
- How does it feel to represent these situations, to write about them and to read this out loud to the group?

9.8 ASSIGNMENT 6: Self-Portrait—Four Sentences

Make an art work with 'self-portrait' as the theme.
It does not necessarily have to be a portrait of a face. It may also be an abstract design, or three-dimensional, or something else, it's entirely up to you.
Take your inspiration from one or more of the following sentences (*Art magazine Dada theme issue 'self-portrait' 2004*):

- I am who I am.
- I am more than what you see.
- I don't just show everything.
- Maybe I am only what you see.

OBJECT:

Gaining insight into how you see yourself.
Gaining insight into your contacts with others.
Sharing your personal theme, 'self-image /self-portrait', with the group.

MATERIALS:

Free choice.

INDIVIDUALLY in the Group

EXPLANATORY NOTES:

People may combine two sentences if they wish.
In the follow-up discussion, group members may first react to art works made by others. What is there to see?

EVALUATION:

- In the follow-up discussion, have clients go back to the four sentences.
- Which sentence said the most to you?
- What did you do with it?
- What sort of effect does what the maker says about the work have on his or her contact with the group?
- Do group members recognise you in the portrait you made?

9.9 ASSIGNMENT 7: The Four Elements

In this assignment, the four elements (earth, water, fire, air) are the starting point. Each of these elements stands for something different. Try to identify the feelings aroused in you by these elements and make a choice on this basis.
From these elements, choose:
1. one which is very familiar to you, with which you can identify on the basis of who you are and your own personal history.
2. one which is less familiar to you, in relation to which you would like to develop or are already developing.

Give shape to both of these in a personal way, either as two separate representations, or joined in combined works or in a single expressive work.

OBJECT:

Acquiring insight into personal themes and your personal process.
Making a connection between design, use of materials and the appeal of the various elements and personal themes.

MATERIALS:

Free choice.

INDIVIDUALLY in the Group

EXPLANATORY NOTES:

In working with this assignment, encourage the use of different materials that may be suited to the theme.
If you ask clients to work abstractly, this lessens the chance that the work they produce is stereotyped or hackneyed.

Earth: ground, basis, calm, stable
Water: emotion, flowing, streams
Fire: passion, fiery spirit, conflict
Air: fleeting, thoughts, light

EVALUATION:

- What was it like to work on this? (the process of working)
- What is there to see? (the description of the work)
- What personal significance, or personal substance, does it have? (interpretation)
- Do the group members recognise these aspects for the person who made it?

If the story diverges too much from the actual work, ask questions in order to draw attention back to the work.

9.10 ASSIGNMENT 8: Lines—Circle—Human Figure

The therapist instructs:
'Using oil pastels, draw step by step on a sheet of paper (50–65 cm):
- 4 horizontal lines, it's up to you where and how you place them, straight, curved, crooked or tight and snug,
- 3 vertical lines,
- a circle,
- a human figure.

Using Ecoline liquid watercolours, develop this composition in any way you like'.

OBJECT:

Working within a structure in which you surrender to the situation.
Becoming aware of how you assign meaning.
Becoming aware of your own patterns, emotions.

MATERIALS:

Oil pastels and Ecoline liquid watercolours.

INDIVIDUALLY in the Group

EXPLANATORY NOTES:

The therapist provides a directive approach for carrying out this assignment step by step. The idea is for clients not to devote too much attention to thinking about the assignment or to their interpretation of the final result. It is important that group members allow themselves to be led and are open to surprises and spontaneity. The use of the combination of oil pastels and watercolours may give rise to investigation of and experimentation with the materials.

EVALUATION:

Before the follow-up discussion, clients may first write down titles for their own work and that of the others. In that case, first the group members read out their titles for work 1, and the maker reads out his or hers after that. In this way, everyone gives an initial reaction to the work of others and to its expressiveness. They look closely at each others' work, and the maker gains insight into what the work evokes in others (this offers a view of the blind spot in the Johari window: what you do not see but others do, or the facade: what you see but others do not).

- What was it like to do this assignment?
- What was it like to be given a structure in the form of lines, a shape and a figure? Could you accept this and work with it, or what took place during the process?
- Do you recognise certain themes in the image that come forward here? Were you already consciously focused on this while working, or did you see the significance later?
- What did you think of the materials, the combination of materials?

9.11 ASSIGNMENT 9: Six Basic Emotions

Start from six of the basic emotions: **happiness, sadness, anger, fear, surprise and disgust.**

Part 1: Choose an emotion that is close to you right now, and try to portray it in the act of drawing. Do not use recognisable images or symbols, but choose a movement, colour or line that is appropriate to your feeling. Continue in this way for a little while.

Part 2: Now, work on the basis of the same emotion but in a symbolic manner, or with recognisable images.
What is the difference?

OBJECT:

Reflecting on the feeling it gives you, investigating: What am I actually feeling?
Discovering the differences between various ways of approaching the emotion.

MATERIALS:

Pastels, oil pastels.

INDIVIDUALLY in the Group

EXPLANATORY NOTES:

The difference between part 1 and part 2 can be found in the more intellectual or more intuitive approach to the emotion.

EVALUATION:

- Which of these manners brings you in closer contact with the emotion?
- Is that pleasant or not so pleasant for you?
- How do you usually deal with emotions, and is this manner more suited to the first or the second manner of dealing with them?
- What else would you like to do on the basis of this assignment?

9.12 ASSIGNMENT 10: Black Ink Monsters

Splash or spatter India ink spots on paper; if you like, use a paintbrush, sponge, etc. Use your imagination to make one or more monsters in this way. You can amplify the effect by drawing or sticking on eyes, and by developing the surroundings using black felt pen, liquid watercolours and snippets of paper that show a pattern or design.

This can be done both individually and in a group. In a group, the sheets of paper can be joined together to make one long strip, so that you can work together on the edges where your sheet of paper and your neighbour's meet. You can also choose to work on a single large sheet of paper.

OBJECT:

Working with chance, in which you surrender to the situation of the moment.
Using imagination.
Working with the emotion of aggression, symbolised by the black monster.
Becoming aware of how you assign meaning.
Becoming aware of your own patterns, emotions.

MATERIALS:

India ink, paintbrush, sponge, dip pen, various shades of liquid watercolours, bits of paper with a pattern or design, eyes with adhesive backing.

INDIVIDUAL/GROUP

EXPLANATORY NOTES:

Could also be used to make a comic strip (have the monsters say something in a text balloon, make a story with a sequence of several pictures).

The therapist provides a directive approach for carrying out this assignment step by step. The idea is not for clients to spend much time thinking about the assignment or making their own interpretation of the final result. It is important that they allow themselves to be led and leave room for surprises and spontaneity.

The combination of materials may form a reason to investigate and experiment with the materials.

EVALUATION:

- What was it like to do this assignment?
- What was it like to make spots with ink? Could you accept this and work with it, or what took place during the process?
- Did you manage to make monsters in this way? Are your monsters dangerous, aggressive, or are they cute, dopey little things? Did you give the monsters any particular expression?
- Were you consciously focused on this while working, or did you only see the significance later?
- What did you think of the materials, the combination of materials?

9.13 ASSIGNMENT 11: Above and Below the Surface

Draw a line on a sheet of paper to represent the surface.
Draw what you let others see (this comes above the surface) and what you put below it, things you don't let others see (they stay below the surface).

OBJECT:

Becoming aware of and gaining insight into your own emotions.
Learning to communicate about emotions, becoming more open.

MATERIALS:

Black ink, reed pen, dip pen, paintbrush, water, liquid watercolours.

INDIVIDUALLY in the Group

EXPLANATORY NOTES:

This assignment invites clients to show more than they usually do. It allows them to practise being more open, communicating more about their own feelings, and how to regulate emotions by expressing them or by keeping them 'below the surface'.

EVALUATION:

- What was it like to work with the theme of above and below the surface? What sorts of things did you encounter?
- Tell something about how you experienced this.
- Do the group members recognise this as something that is well suited to you? (question for the group members)

9.14 ASSIGNMENT 12: The Wall

Give everyone a sheet of brick paper.

Let this paper inspire you and use it to make your own work.

What would you like to do with it, what could you do with it? What kind of feelings does this arouse in you? Use this inspiration to make something personal.

OBJECT:

Becoming aware of, gaining insight into and learning to deal with walls in the symbolic sense of the word, such as boundaries, resistance or restrictions.

MATERIALS:

Pre-printed brick paper, plus free choice of materials.

INDIVIDUALLY in the Group

EXPLANATORY NOTES:

In this assignment, it is interesting to learn what the brick paper arouses in clients and what they do with the response it evokes: is the response used to give form to the emotion, or do clients fight it or repress it.

EVALUATION:

- What sorts of feelings did the brick paper arouse in you at first? What did you do with this?
- Describe how you arrived at the work you made.
- What do we see in the work?
- What theme or themes does it show?
- Do other recognise this about you? (question for the group members)

9.15 ASSIGNMENT 13: Timeline of Your Life

Make your own lifeline on paper. It starts when you were born and it continues up to today.
On this line, show how your life has unfolded thus far. This may mean that different periods look very different to each other. The line can have colours, it can be thick, thin, irregular or smooth. You can also represent events on the line by portraying them by means of form, line or colour.

OBJECT:

Learning to accept and to use the emotions aroused by making your lifeline.
Gaining insight into your own behaviour pattern in dealing with difficult emotions.

MATERIALS:

Pastels, paper.

INDIVIDUALLY in the Group

EXPLANATORY NOTES:

If you like, you can point out that it does not actually have to be a timeline, so that clients can look for more expressive ways of putting their life on paper.
It is possible that two sessions will be needed for this assignment, depending on how quickly clients work and on the breadth and depth intended by you as the therapist.
In this assignment, emphasis does not necessarily lie on the content of the work, but more on how clients deal with emotions; whether they can accept and deal with difficult emotions. The lifeline of many of these clients is often marked by traumatic experiences.

EVALUATION:

- Can you tell us something about your lifeline?
- What does making and telling about your lifeline arouse in you, how does it make you feel?
- What is it like to look at it now, with some distance?
- How do you deal with the emotion(s) it has aroused? What can you do so that you will be able to handle or accept these emotions more readily? Is there something that you are doing differently now than you did a while ago?

9.16 ASSIGNMENT 14: Timeline of Your Life (Continued)

Choose a contrast from the lifeline that you made last time.
Develop this further.

OBJECT:

Gaining insight into polarities in your own person or your own history.
Bringing together extremes in a single representation, promoting integrative capacities.

MATERIALS:

Free choice.

INDIVIDUALLY in the Group

EXPLANATORY NOTES:

Another subsequent assignment might be to choose a positive and/or a negative moment in the lifeline and to develop that in a new work.

EVALUATION:

- What is the contrast you chose?
- How did you develop this? What was it like to work on this?
- What do you find striking about it?
- Does this contrast have personal significance for you?
- Do you recognise this contrast as fitting to two sides of yourself?

9.17 ASSIGNMENT 15: Black and White Tearing Exercise

Take a large sheet of white paper (50 × 65 cm) and a sheet of black paper half that size (32.5 × 50 cm).

Using your finger, poke a hole in the middle of the black paper and starting from the hole, tear out a shape from the middle of the black paper. Leave the edges of the paper whole. Put the torn bits aside. Then paste the original piece of black paper (32.5 × 65 cm) on half of the white sheet of paper, so that one half stays white and the other half is black with a white hole or with white holes.

Now, paste the pieces of black paper that you tore out on to the white half. The idea is to use them to make a black animal. The white holes on the black half will also form an animal. Use pastels to work out these animals.

In our discussion later, a dialogue between these two animals will be invented.

OBJECT:

Participating.
Investigating contrasts or polarities in yourself.
Developing insight into polarities.

MATERIALS:

Per person, one sheet of white paper (50 × 65 cm) and a sheet of black paper half that size (32.5 × 60 cm).
Pastels.
Black felt pen or fine liner and white marker or white chalk.

INDIVIDUALLY in the Group

EXPLANATORY NOTES:

This assignment is based on the polarising effect between the white and the black. The black animal readily becomes the bad, sullen, grumbling or aggressive animal, while the white animal is often seen as the innocent, cheerful, adorable and good animal.

The specific polarity this contains may be recognised as a client's own personal theme. Even if this is not recognised, it is in any case an assignment in which playful elements are key and it has a fairly high level of surprise because no one knows exactly where it is leading, and because clients must continue fantasising in order to turn the bits and pieces into animals.

EVALUATION:

- What was it like to do this assignment? How did you feel about the fact that you did not really know where it was going?
- Can you tell us something about your two animals? What sort of character do they exhibit?
- If one of them were to say something to the other, which of them would say something?

- What would it say? (Write this on the work in a text balloon.)
- What would the other animal say back? (Write this down too.)
- Do you recognise the conflict between these two animals? You might see it as two sides of yourself having a conversation or an argument.

9.18 ASSIGNMENT 16: House of Emotions

Design your own house where basic emotions live, such as anger, fear, surprise, interest, guilt/shame, sadness, happiness and disgust. You can give them all a place in the rooms, or they can have a place inside or outside the house. The house symbolises you.

Using lines, shapes and colour, develop the emotions in an expressive manner. Decide for yourself where you will place emotions, how much space a particular emotion takes up and perhaps which emotions will be close together. Give each room a colour that is appropriate to the way you experience the emotion.

Think about and be aware of why you put the emotion in that place, and why you represent it in that way (where have you put it, is it large or small, familiar, intense, repressed, far away or in the foreground, what colour, what is next to it, do you want to add some details, etc.).

OBJECT:

An exercise in thinking about yourself and your own emotions.
Gaining insight into the dynamics of the basic emotions and the relationships between them.

MATERIALS:

Pastels, paper, format of your own choice.

INDIVIDUALLY in the Group

EXPLANATORY NOTES:

Perhaps the situation in the house can be worked out by asking them to start a dialogue: 'What do the emotions say to each other?', or perhaps their relationship can be investigated by asking them about, or focusing on, the hierarchy.

EVALUATION:

- Tell something about your house that you just made and your reasons for doing it that way.
- What emotions are represented in abundance, and what emotions have little presence?
- What can you say about how you placed the various emotions?

9.19 ASSIGNMENT 17: Two Stones—Holding on and Letting Go

A number of stones are lying on the table. Clients choose two stones and put them in front of themselves. We start with an imagination exercise (perhaps preceded by a brief introduction, if clients are not used to this type of exercise). They all push their chairs back a bit from the table so that there is enough room for everyone to sit, and so that they can all concentrate and are not distracted by the others around them.

The therapist instructs:
'Sit down and relax in your chair, put your legs next to each other, straight, feet on the floor aligned with your hips. If you like, you may close your eyes. If you prefer, just let your eyes rest on a neutral point in front of you. Sit up straight, don't lean on the chair back or the table, keep your back straight and imagine that your head is being held up by a thread through the top of your head... Your arms rest quietly on your

legs. Focus your attention on your breathing. Is your breathing calm ... is it fast or slow, are your breaths at the top of your chest, or deeper, reaching your abdomen? Breathe in and out deeply and try to let your breaths go deeper. Don't be distracted by sounds you may hear around you, just observe and let go of them. Focus your attention on your head and the muscles in your face, try to relax them, or if you like, first tense them and then relax them ... Focus your attention on your neck and feel whether you can relax here too ... Go to your shoulders, feel the tension that may be there, tense up and then relax ... Go to your arms and your hands, tense up and relax ... Focus your attention on your back and your abdomen, feel the muscles and feel how you carry yourself, let this tension relax too ... Go to your legs, your knees, your lower legs and your ankles, tense up and relax ... Now feel how your feet are flat on the floor, and imagine that you can let any tension you might still feel disappear into the floor ...'

'Now turn your thoughts to the last few months ... What have you had to let go of in the last few months... .what did you want to leave behind, what did you have to leave behind? This could be just about anything. Maybe it was a certain habit, a certain behaviour or an expectation that you had. Perhaps it was a person, or several people. Try to form a picture of this in your mind that is as clear as possible. What do you see? You can convert it into a symbol. What symbol represents best what you see? What colours do you see? Are the shapes round or angular, with pointy corners?'

'Now turn your thoughts to the near future ... What do you want to focus on in the coming period? What do you want to hold on to? Maybe it is something that you have discovered, or have experienced ... What is important for you to hold on to? Try to form a clear picture of this for yourself. What do you see? You can convert this into a symbol as well. What symbol represents best what you see? What colours do you see? Are the shapes round or angular, with pointy corners? ... Look at this image once more, and then leave it for what it is for the time being'.

'Bring your attention back in the room; where are you now? Do you hear sounds? When you are ready, open your eyes ... take your time'.

'Now take your two stones. Represent what you want to let go of on one stone, and what you want to hold on to on the other stone. Try to keep your attention focused on yourself and not to talk to others'.

OBJECT:

Coming in contact with and gaining insight into your own experiences, your feelings of mourning and/or letting go.
Learning to focus on and hold on to what you want.
Showing the group how you give shape to personal experiences and making the group a partner in your experiences and feelings.

MATERIALS:

2 stones (beach stones) per person, acrylic paints and thin paintbrushes.
Perhaps a hair dryer to speed up the drying process.

INDIVIDUALLY in the Group

EXPLANATORY NOTES:

This assignment is contraindicated if a client is psychotic or has a borderline psychosis, or could decompensate. The fear of losing control and being overwhelmed by emotions may be too great, in which case the assignment might only increase anxiety. It has been my experience that anxious participants can sometimes benefit when they do not actually take part, but simply observe. This is because something speaks to them or is aroused in them, something that can be developed in their expressive work.

EVALUATION:

- How did you experience this exercise; did the images come to mind easily (or not), did the process of arousing images stop somewhere (or not), and what could be the reason for this?
- What feelings arose in you?
- What do you want to take with you/what do you want to hold on to?

<u>Homework assignment</u>
The therapist instructs:

'Take both stones with you. The idea is to give the stone you want to hold on to a nice place of its own, in a place where you will see it regularly and can pick it up, hold it. Within two days, you take the other stone, showing what you want to leave behind, or must leave behind, and you leave it wherever you want, consciously paying attention to what you do ... you can put it in the ground, throw it into the water, it makes no difference as long as you find a suitable place for this stone. If you find this very difficult, it may be too early to make such a choice. Decide for yourself what is within reach'.
At the next session, we will come back to this and the therapist will ask: What did you decide to do with the stones, and did you do just that? How did it go?

9.20 ASSIGNMENT 18: Elevenie

Everyone takes a pen and paper. Step by step, we will write an Eleven Tree. This is a short poem consisting of eleven words in the following structure:

1
2 3
4 5 6
7 8 9 10
11

After that, everyone will read their poems and draw a picture that suits or strengthens the atmosphere of the poem.

The poem is part of the picture; the literal text will be in the picture in such a way that the picture and the words support and strengthen each other.

OBJECT:

Becoming aware of and giving shape to feelings and thoughts.

MATERIALS:

Pen, A4 paper, A3 and A2 paper.
Flat surface, materials: paint, chalk, Ecoline liquid watercolours, translucent paper, glue.
Optional: stencil letters.

INDIVIDUALLY in the Group

EXPLANATORY NOTES:

An elevenie is a very simple poetic form that allows you to play with words and to take poetic freedom, even people who never write poems. People are often surprised by the result.

EVALUATION:

- How did you experience this assignment?
- What do you think of the result?

9.21 ASSIGNMENT 19: Human Figure and Geometric Shape

Make a human figure from clay. And make a geometric shape, a sphere, a cube, a pyramid or some other shape. Combine these to form a single work. This means that the two parts are literally placed in a relationship with each other.

Investigate what is important about both parts; how do you want the human figure or the shape to look, what size will they be (large or small), how will you finish the surface, what relationship do you want it to show and what do you want to it to express?

OBJECT:

Separating observing features of images from personal meaning or interpretation.
Observing features, contrasts, differences and similarities in the image.
Gaining insight into the personal meaning of the work or insight into your own patterns.

MATERIALS:

Clay in various colours, clay-working tools.

INDIVIDUALLY in the Group

EXPLANATORY NOTES:

This assignment is useful for learning to separate more objective observations from subjective experience and interpretation, and to identify personal themes on that basis. The outcome of this assignment may result in another work.
One way of dealing with the follow-up discussion is asking each other questions, as an exercise in separating what you see and what it means.

EVALUATION:

The initial focus is on simply observing expressive features:

- What do you find striking about the work?
- What expressive aspects are the most striking?

- What characterises the human figure and what characterises the geometric shape?
- How are the two parts related?

After that, the focus is on personal meaning:

- Can you give it a title?
- What might you like to do with it now?
- Do you recognise the theme present in the work as related to you?
- Is the theme connected to your treatment goals and if so, how?

9.22 ASSIGNMENT 20: Emotion Island—Map

Make a drawing of an island seen from above. Express your inner view, your personal emotions, on the basis of this 'atlas' of an island or island group—for example, different landscape elements, what goes with what and where you want to put it.

To encourage associations, first go around the group and have each person name something. If you like, they can also think up names. The names can be written on the drawing close to the towns, lakes, rivers and areas on the map. A name could express a relationship between an emotion and a landscape element. For example, the desert of boredom.

OBJECT:

Recognising and giving shape to emotions.
Investigating relationships between various emotions.

MATERIALS:

Pastels, paper, format of your choice.

INDIVIDUALLY in the Group

EXPLANATORY NOTES:

A book such as the *Atlas of Emotions* can serve as inspiration. This has some disadvantages: the emotional maps are so beautifully elaborated that your own pales in comparison; many things are copied rather than being created by clients.

EVALUATION:

- What was it like to do this assignment?
- What sort of island did you make, and what landscape elements does it have?
- What do the different areas of your island stand for?
- What is striking about the relationships between different regions? What is central, what is at the front, what is out of the way? Does this have significance for you?

9.23 ASSIGNMENT 21: Making Choices

- Take a maximum of 10 minutes to select pictures from magazines that say something to you, that may affect you in an emotional sense or be of interest to you (no texts).
- Put away the magazines.
- Cut or tear everything off the selected pictures that is not important.
- Put all the pictures in front of you on the table and choose three of them.
- Go round the group and have everyone explain his or her choice.
- Using two L-shaped white corners of paper, make a choice by placing them on the pictures like a passepartout. Use the part of the pictures that inspires you the most. Based on this cutaway, make an expressive work in which an enlargement of this image is used as the starting point. Use your creative freedom to add your own twist, to find your own design.

OBJECT:

Making choices.
Investigating emotions: exploring, recognising and acknowledging emotions.
Recognising and naming what appeals to you, touches you.

MATERIALS:

Magazines, newspapers, scissors, 2 white paper L-shapes which can serve as a frame when they overlap each other in mirror image.
Drawing and/or painting materials, large white sheet of paper, format of choice.

INDIVIDUALLY in the Group

EXPLANATORY NOTES:

The instructions state that texts may not be selected. This is meant to encourage clients to look at images and aspects of them. Texts very readily draw all attention to themselves.

EVALUATION:

- Were you able to make choices and concentrate on them as you went along?
- What appealed to you, what touched you in the pictures and what did you do with them? What did you get from this?
- What does it feel like to look at your work afterwards?

9.24 ASSIGNMENT 22: Emergence of a Painting

Choose acrylic paint in several colours. Using these colours and a coarse paintbrush, cover the entire surface of the paper with spots, blotches, stripes or large dots until it is completely covered (20 minutes). It is not supposed to look like anything. You can mix the colours as much as you like.

After this, take time to look at the background and set to work with a fine paintbrush, so that a picture emerges from the spots. Let yourself be guided by what you can see and what it evokes in you (15 minutes).

OBJECT:

Allowing a picture to emerge (discovering it), possibly also gaining insight into more subconscious perception.
Participating by sharing associations relating to material, form and colour.

MATERIALS:

Acrylic paint, coarse and fine paintbrush, cardboard or paper, format 50×65 cm or larger.

INDIVIDUALLY in the Group

EXPLANATORY NOTES:

To stimulate the imagination, the session could start with a warming-up exercise.

EVALUATION:

- What was it like to fill the entire surface with paint without making it look like anything?
- What did you see in it later? How did you continue working on it?
- What does the picture show now? What does it say about you?
- What does it feel like when you look at it now?

9.25 ASSIGNMENT 23: Self-Portrait, Inside and Out

Make two self-portraits, one as you often feel inside and one as you usually show yourself to the outside world. Do this by making a diptych on which your picture of yourself from head to shoulders is the starting point.

OBJECT:

Acquiring self-insight.
Becoming aware of the difference between inside and outside and the effect this has on communication.

MATERIALS:

Drawing or painting materials, paper or cardboard, perhaps a mirror.

INDIVIDUALLY in the Group

EXPLANATORY NOTES:

This assignment can also be carried out by making a plaster of Paris mask and painting it both inside and out based on the theme. The mask can be made from a real face, but this is often felt to be constricting or oppressive. One solution is to use a clay shape covered with Vaseline as a template.

EVALUATION:

- Describe your two self-portraits in terms of how you made them and how you arrived at these choices.
- Do the group members recognise the inside and outside of the person? (question for the group members)
- What effect does this inside/outside theme have on contact with others? What did you learn from this; when does it bother you?

9.26 Evaluation Form for Emotion Regulation

Name:

What emotion did you experience the most strongly before, during and after working on your art work?
(did it feel good, exciting, gripping or did you feel sad)

Did you notice any physical changes or observations?
(what did you feel in your body, for example: a lump in your throat, tense shoulders, etc.)

What was your body language like?
(what sort of feeling did you radiate, were you relaxed in your work, did you look irritated, etc.)

How did you interpret working expressively and the work you made?
(describe the way you felt about it, your thoughts about it)

How do you feel in retrospect/what after-effect does it have for you?

What did you say about it in our follow-up discussion, and are you satisfied with that?

10
Interpersonal Effectiveness Module

10.1 Summary of Interpersonal Effectiveness Theory

The skills in this module have much in common with skills that are learned in assertiveness training or conflict training. They are effective strategies in asking for what you need, being able to say no and dealing with conflicts. In this context, effective means achieving the desired changes, maintaining a relationship and maintaining your self-respect. The object is to stand up for your own wishes, goals and opinions in a way in which other people take them seriously. In the process, interpersonal relationships and self-respect are not damaged, but reinforced.

Generally speaking, most people have reasonable to good interpersonal skills. Often, problems arise in specific situations: deep-rooted convictions and uncontrollable emotional reactions get in the way of actually applying the skills they have learned.

People who have difficulty with emotion regulation often hesitate between avoiding a conflict and winding up in a huge confrontation. In this regard, not what the situation calls for but a person's emotional state generally determines the response, which can cause serious

S. Haeyen, *Art Therapy and Emotion Regulation Problems*,
https://doi.org/10.1007/978-3-319-96773-8_10

problems in relationships with others and in a person's own relationship with himself or herself.

Interpersonal Effectiveness means:

Attend to relationships

The ability to restore relationships is much more important than preventing even the tiniest rift or fissure.

Balance priorities and demands

This equilibrium is the first task in structuring a person's life so that it does not become too empty or too full. People who are overwhelmed or overstretched need to work out the most important priorities and demands and then say no to less important ones. Some people, on the other hand, have too few priorities and demands. In that case, it is important for them to structure the demands made of them and to accept the more important ones.

Balance what you want to do and what you should do

A healthy lifestyle requires some degree of equilibrium between what a person wants to do and what he or she should do. How does this look in a person's life, and how does that person want to bring their life back in balance?

Develop mastery and self-respect

A person must do things that, although difficult, must be done, things that form a challenge. By attending to their own values and convictions and by taking pride in dealing with difficult situations, a person develops self-respect. Mastery is getting up after a fall: the fall itself is not important. Interpersonal situations are often the most difficult to master. You can learn mastery by practising interpersonal skills.

Objects of interpersonal effectiveness

Effectiveness focused on a goal

Making sure you achieve your goal in a certain situation. Learning to deal with frustration and to accept reality is closely bound up with interpersonal skills.

Effectiveness focused on a relationship

Building and maintaining a good relationship. The object is to maintain or even improve an interpersonal relationship while also trying to achieve your goals. Using interpersonal skills will not only strengthen relationships, but it will also increase your chance of gaining interpersonal and social appreciation.

Effectiveness focused on self-respect

Retaining or improving self-respect and self-esteem. Feeling good about yourself, retaining and improving this feeling and respecting your values and convictions while working to achieve your goals. This means doing what you consider ethical and what makes you feel competent. A person will have a hard time believing he is nice if he continually takes advantage of others; he may get what he wants, but it is at the expense of his self-respect.

Questions: When did you do something that caused your self-respect to decline? When did you feel that your self-respect had grown? What are aspects on which you need to improve your skills?

Encouraging words and effective skills are important for interpersonal effectiveness.

Encouraging comments for interpersonal effectiveness

These are things people say to themselves to give themselves permission, to ask for what they want or need, to say no and to act effectively. There are two types of encouraging or supportive statements: statements that give you the courage to conduct yourself effectively, and statements that help you to prepare for a situation, to be effective and to focus on what works.

In this module, a person's own statements are examined and they learn to use supportive statements.

Effective skills

Skills for achieving goals, for maintaining relationships and preserving self-respect: asking for things, making requests, engaging in conversations; saying no, withstanding pressure, sticking to a position or point of view.

To achieve these skills, it is important that you learn to observe and describe interpersonal situations and to practise skills. This is how people learn, for example, how to ask for something and to refuse something in a way that is suitable. It may be appropriate to make a request in one situation, while in another situation the same request may not be the least bit appropriate. The same applies to refusing requests. This is an important skill. Learning to be clear and concise is important, as is learning how to talk about your thoughts—for example, about self-harm or suicide—without giving another person the feeling of being manipulated.

Inhibiting factors

Factors that decrease interpersonal effectiveness are a lack of skills, worrisome thoughts, emotions, indecisiveness or hesitation, and the surroundings. Emotional reactions may be based on earlier experiences, but also on myths that are wrongly held to be true. Myths can be refuted by using logical counterarguments or through corrective experiences.

10.2 Multidisciplinary Relationships in the Various Aspects of Treatment

Dialectical Behaviour Therapy (DBT)
Module: Interpersonal Effectiveness Skills

Emotional dysregulation, particularly anger and difficulty in expressing it, easily leads to confusion in relationships. Social skills are needed in order to establish relationships.

Skills:
- effective strategies in asking for what a person needs
- being able to say no
- dealing with conflicts

Skills training	Psycho-education: weigh up the interests of achieving the goal (1), maintaining the relationship (2) and retaining self-respect (3) Behavioural analysis and examining motives: What interest takes priority? Role-playing
Homework	Complete the behavioural analysis form; discuss the effects of various choices
Basic group	Unstructured group in which the focus may be, for example, patterns in previous relationships

Art therapy	Investigating group interactions and practising different behaviour—for example, learning to have fun or kid around with each other, learning to deal with conflict using the materials; group painting; variations in shared assignments. Art therapy as tangible evidence of interaction and as something to reflect on. Direct link between action and reflection creates a practice area. Practising with boundaries (of yourself, of others, of the materials). Representing experiences with interactions; how you view the self and the other, sociogram
Music therapy	Each assignment devotes attention to the object, to the relationship and to self-respect. Exercises for setting boundaries, making contact and learning to allow yourself to do things. For example, playing the djembé (African drum), where everyone has their own rhythm or task. Basic rhythm, counter-rhythm, beginning, ending, etc. Learning to maintain your own position while continuing to make contact and seek continuity
Psychomotor therapy	Asking for help or support while retaining autonomy (e.g. in an exercise with your eyes closed), acknowledging or setting boundaries (e.g. taking a controlled approach, defending your own territory), dealing with opposing interests (e.g. in forms of movement). Forms of therapy focused on discovering how much space you need
Sociotherapy opening/ closing the daily session/ surroundings	During the daily closing session, agreeing that it is a good idea to call a friend, something you have been planning to do for days During the social reintegration forum, making a plan containing concrete steps on how you deal with social contacts. Giving each other feedback. How do you handle conflict?

10.3 ASSIGNMENT 1: What Are You Looking for in Contacts with Others and/or in Working with Materials?

Choose a material that is one of your favourites as well as another material that is the opposite or not one of your favourites.
Join these materials in an art work.

OBJECT:

Identifying your own behavioural patterns and needs.
Reflecting on handling boundaries, conflict.

MATERIALS:

2 materials that are complete opposites (free choice).

INDIVIDUALLY in the Group

EXPLANATORY NOTES:

It is important that there are a wide range and a large variety of materials to choose from.

EVALUATION:

- Describe what appeals to you in the first material and what you do not like about the other one.
- What does the material arouse in you; what are you looking for when you work with materials?
- Did you spend a different amount of time on one material or the other?
- How do you work with the material? How does this process take place?
- Is there a similarity?
- What do you think of the expressive work you made?

10.4 ASSIGNMENT 2: Sociogram

Make a representation of you and your most important relationships. In how you represent this, make it clear what relationship you have with these people. Who is close to you, who is further away, how can you show the nature of the different relationships?

You do not have to actually draw people, but if you do, the drawings do not need to resemble them. You can represent people and relationships abstractly by making them a particular colour or shape, for example.

OBJECT:

Gaining awareness and insight into important relationships.

MATERIALS:

Paper 50 × 65 cm, drawing materials.

INDIVIDUALLY in the Group

EXPLANATORY NOTES:

In the follow-up discussion, certain things may come forward—for example, that a person has very many relationships, or very few, that certain people are conspicuously absent, or that some people find their family very important, whereas others find friends very important. This can also be linked to goals in relation to a person's social network.

EVALUATION:

- How did you draw the sociogram? Who is who and what place is occupied by the relationships?
- What is the nature of these relationships?

- What interpersonal skills play a role in these relationships?
- What conflicts (if any) do they involve?
- Are certain persons represented at a striking distance, or extremely close by?

10.5 ASSIGNMENT 3: Working in Pairs—Postcards

Before starting, the group members reflect on the goals they have formulated for themselves in relation to interpersonal skills. They are asked with which of the group members they could best work on their goals. Have them form pairs on this basis.

Each person individually chooses one card or picture from a pile of postcards or magazine pages (with nature photographs, for example). Each person chooses what appeals to him or her.

As a result, each pair has two cards or pictures. The pair determines how they will use these pictures as the basis for one joint expressive work. The intention is to work together and to produce a single work. Together, the two persons choose an idea that is based on both pictures, for example, by using the picture on one card and the colours on the other one. The two decide between themselves how much of one picture and how much of the other will be used. The ratio does not necessarily have to be fifty-fifty.

Stress the fact that, in choosing and in working together on their representation, they must focus on their interpersonal effectiveness goals.

OBJECT:

Working together: making choices, learning to consult with each other and together arriving at a shared result.
Being assertive to achieve what you want.
Conflict management.
Giving and receiving positive feedback.

MATERIALS:

Free choice, to be determined by the two persons jointly.

IN PAIRS

EXPLANATORY NOTES:

EVALUATION:

- What appealed to you in the card you chose?
- How was your working relationship? Which of you was more the leader, which one more the follower, in making decisions? Who chose the picture, who chose the materials?
- Does the work show that it was made by two different persons, or does it look like one person made it?
- In the work you made together, do you recognise what appealed to you in the card you chose?
- In retrospect, is the work in line with your wishes, or did it become something completely different when the two of you worked together? In other words, does it feel enough as if it is yours? What percentage is yours?
- Did you practise working towards a goal that you set for yourself to achieve greater interpersonal effectiveness? What made this happen, or not happen?

- What did you enjoy about how your partner presented himself or herself in your work together? Tell your partner what you valued in working together.
- What about yourself are you satisfied with?

10.6 ASSIGNMENT 4: Emotion and Collaboration

Everyone draws a card with an emotion on it. Investigate for yourself how this emotion feels, what attitude you adopt, how you react verbally and non-verbally when you feel it.

Together with one or two others who drew the same card, make a work based on the emotion in which you try to express the emotion so that, when others see it, they will know what emotion your work refers to. In making this work, you make use of the power of expression of the materials themselves.

OBJECT:

Exploring, recognising and acknowledging emotions.
Exploring working together.

MATERIALS:

Cards with various emotions (afraid, angry, happy, sad). Free choice of materials.

IN PAIRS OR THREESOMES

EXPLANATORY NOTES:

Suggested variation: Working in pairs, the first person draws an emotion card and does not tell the other person what it says. The two of them set to work and the person who drew the card will try to put the emotion across to the other person by means of the expressive work, therefore also non-verbally. Optionally, a few other persons can observe and note what they see in the way of facial expressions, use of materials, forms and colours.

EVALUATION:

- Were you able to express the emotion?
- Was a particular emotion more difficult than another one?
- How did you use the materials?
- Were you able to give the materials emotional expressiveness?
- Do you know the emotion well that you worked out?
- What was it like, working together with someone else on this?

10.7 ASSIGNMENT 5: Three Sheets of Paper, Working Towards Each Other

Each pair of participants joins three sheets of paper of 50 × 65 cm on the reverse using sticky tape, to make one long sheet of paper. Each of you may choose four colours of paint to work with; put them on a palette.

Each of you starts working on one of the short sides of the long paper. The first sheet on each side is the individual part, where you may do whatever you want in the way you choose. The sheet in the middle is the shared part, where you decide together what will happen there. You must work non-verbally!

OBJECT:

Experiencing differences in and gaining insight into working individually and working together.
Learning to coordinate your work and to work together.

MATERIALS:

3 sheets of paper of 50 × 65 cm per pair.
Paints, brushes.

IN PAIRS

EXPLANATORY NOTES:

In this assignment, interpersonal effectiveness means finding a balance between attention to your own part, your own manner of working, and attention to the part you do together, where it is important to coordinate your work and work together.

EVALUATION:

- How did you work on the individual part?
- In the first part, were you able to stay concentrated on yourself? While working on your individual part, were you keeping an eye on what your partner was doing at the same time?
- How was the transition to the middle part?
- What was it like to coordinate your work, to work together? What did you encounter in this regard?
- What do you think of the result?

10.8 ASSIGNMENT 6: Plaster of Paris Hands

Working in pairs, each of you puts a plaster cast all around the other person's hand. This process demands preparation, attention and great care. The idea is to make a hand-shaped cast of each group member.
After that, a group work can be made by bringing all these hands together (e.g. in a mobile, a composition or by placing them in specific surroundings).

OBJECT:

Learning to work together.
Giving and receiving attention.
Practising with closeness and intimacy.

MATERIALS:

Pre-cut pieces of a plaster cast, scissors, bucket with lukewarm water, Vaseline to rub on your hands before starting.

IN PAIRS

EXPLANATORY NOTES:

Putting a plaster cast on each other's hand is about touching and being in direct physical contact while working together. Concentration, care and attention play an important role. You either lead the way or undergo the process. Because the touching aspect is so direct, it is also about intimacy.

Combining the hands into a group work is primarily about collaboration, group roles and social and/or assertive behaviour.

Optionally, hands can be plastered together, but this requires more support, and it is more complicated to get the plaster off later.
A plaster cast can be put on other body parts as well—on a foot or a face (mask), for instance.
Depending on the size of the group, two sessions may be needed for this assignment.

EVALUATION:

- What was it like to do this assignment?
- What was your experience with it?
- What struck you about it?
- Had you expected to react the way you did?
- What did you think of the result?
- What did you do with the plaster hands to put them together to form a whole?
- What does this say about the group?

10.9 ASSIGNMENT 7: Continuous Garden

Everyone has a large sheet of paper of the same size, and all sheets of paper are put down either horizontally or vertically. Together, group members decide where the horizon is or whether it will be an overhead view.

On the paper you paint your own garden; make it your own place, but be sure that it is connected to the neighbours (how you do this is up to you, perhaps with a hedge, a road, or by continuing colours or shapes from one garden to the next). You work side by side, and the sheets of paper are hung up, adjoining, when everyone is finished.

OBJECT:

Learning to cooperate; adjusting and coordinating while still retaining individuality and autonomy, taking the initiative.

MATERIALS:

Paint and paper, format 50 × 65 cm.

INDIVIDUAL/GROUP

EXPLANATORY NOTES:

Optionally, before starting, a guided fantasy can be provided so that clients can form their own picture of the garden.
It is interesting to see to what extent clients can coordinate and work together without losing sight of their own garden.

Suggested variation: Use a different theme, such as a landscape or a streetscape in which each group member has their own house. The choice of the theme can also be left up to the group.

For the follow-up discussion, the paintings are hung on a wash line. This means that the group members who worked at each end will have only one connecting side, and the others will have two.

EVALUATION:

- Who made the choices for the horizon, who decided whether the paper would be used vertically or horizontally?
- Were you able to concentrate on your own part?
- How did you connect the gardens, or coordinate putting them together (hedge, opening, colours, etc.)?
- Did you have one connecting side or two, and did you think about that beforehand?
- How much did you connect your sheet to others, and how much did you let others connect to your sheet?
- Did you copy elements from someone else's work (colours, composition, light/dark)?
- What does your garden look like; is it a place where you would like to spend time?
- Would you like to be next to someone else's garden?

10.10 ASSIGNMENT 8: Tree and Landscape

Each group member draws a tree without anything else around it, the way he or she feels. When everyone is finished, the trees are cut out. Then the group jointly draws a landscape on a large sheet of paper, with a horizon and various landscape elements. At the end, each of the trees drawn earlier is placed in the landscape.

It is important that group members start at the same time:

- when they start making the surroundings.
- when they start placing the individual items in the surroundings.

OBJECT:

Becoming aware of your present mood, your perception.
Gaining an impression of your own place in the group.
Gaining insight into what you and what others in the group need.
Learning to work together—coordinate, consult, articulate and resolve conflicts.

MATERIALS:

Drawing materials, paper for the individual part 25×45 cm, paper for the group part: depending on group size.

INDIVIDUAL/GROUP

EXPLANATORY NOTES:

Suggested variation:

- Use a different theme, such as jungle animal—jungle; pond animals—pond; house elements—house.
- Everyone first makes the tree and then the landscape is drawn as a joint project, with two group members holding a single charcoal pencil: one of them is the leader, the other follows.

EVALUATION:

- What kind of tree did you make?
- What does this tree say about how you feel?
- Do you have any other associations with the tree; is it a tree that you have seen somewhere before?
- What was it like to make a landscape together after that?
- How was your working relationship?
- Where did you want to put your tree, and where was it placed in the end? Are you satisfied with this? Why did you choose this place?

10.11 ASSIGNMENT 9: Underwater Landscape

Step 1: Using oil pastels, everyone draws their own fish, an existing sort or an imaginary fish, or another kind of underwater animal, but without any surroundings. Then everyone cuts out their drawing.

Step 2: On a large sheet of paper on the table, the group jointly draws an underwater landscape using oil pastels. Somewhere near the top of the sheet, a water line is drawn, and on the bottom of the sheet the bottom of the water. Water plants, stones and objects may be used in the landscape.

Step 3: Everyone takes his or her fish or underwater animal. Together, they are all positioned on the large sheet of paper and pasted there. Everyone decides where they want to put their own drawing.

Step 4: Using Ecoline liquid watercolours in water tints (diluted with lots of water) and sponges, the water is coloured in.

Step 5: Using white paper, a text balloon is made for the fish or underwater animal.
Ask yourself the question: 'If your fish or your animal could talk, what would it say?' It is important to follow the idea that occurs to you first. Then write the text in the text balloon and stick it on the paper.

OBJECT:

In a group situation, providing for your own needs and those of others.
Gaining insight into various positions in the group.
Learning to work together: coordinate, consult, articulate and resolve conflicts.

MATERIALS:

Oil pastel, scissors, Ecoline liquid watercolours in blue and green tints, diluted, sponges, markers.

INDIVIDUAL/GROUP

EXPLANATORY NOTES:

Oil pastel remains visible when the diluted liquid watercolours are applied over it. Light colours in particular are visible and so tiny round white bubbles can be added, air bubbles.

EVALUATION:

- What sort of fish or underwater animal did you make?
- What does it say about you?
- How did you work together to decide on the underwater landscape?
- How did you work together to decide where to place the fish or animals?
- What does the way they are positioned say about you?
- What does your fish or animal say? What does this say about you? Do you recognise this?

10.12 ASSIGNMENT 10: Clay Hut Village

Make long rolls of clay. Cut the rolls into pieces of around 4 cm and using your fingers, make brick shapes out of them. Using these bricks, build your own fantasy house. You may use other materials as well.

When you are finished, the houses everyone has made are placed together so that they form a village. To work this out a bit more, you can make a few more items if you like.

OBJECT:

Devoting attention to your own space and what you need or enjoy having around you.
Starting from your own individuality, making contact with the others and achieving a shared goal.

MATERIALS:

Clay, slats, bases to work on, clay-working tools, natural materials such as twigs, shells, pebbles, cord and small dust rags.

INDIVIDUAL/GROUP

EXPLANATORY NOTES:

If the clay pieces are smoothed together on the inside, the outside of the brick structure can still be seen.

Working with clay bricks takes quite some time. Explain this so that clients don't make large construction plans that cannot be carried out. If you want to spend more time on it, you could divide it over two sessions.

EVALUATION:

- What was it like to make your own house? What is important about the way you designed it?
- How did all of you decide how to place the houses in a village form?
- How does each of you perceive his or her place in the village?
- What does this say about how contact with others takes place in practice? Is it the same here, or is it different? If it is different, why is that?

10.13 ASSIGNMENT 11: Making Contact from Your Personal Space

Place a large sheet of paper on the table and tape it down.
Part 1: Everyone makes an abstract form on the large sheet of paper in a place that stands for 'your own personal space'. Design it any way you want, with your own colour and shape. Decide whether you want to put a fence around it or not and if so, how. Concentrate on yourself. You may not talk to each other.

Part 2: Starting from this space, make contact with one or more others in the group by working on the paper towards the other, using the materials. Here too, work non-verbally. Making contact doesn't just mean drawing a line to another person. See whether you can actually connect.

OBJECT:

Becoming aware of the space you want or need.
Becoming aware of how and with whom you want contact.

MATERIALS:

Large format paper, for example 1×2 metres (depending on the size of the group), soft pastels or oil pastels.

INDIVIDUAL/GROUP

EXPLANATORY NOTES:

Optionally, you could start with a concentration exercise or a work form in which everyone first works on paper of a smaller format and makes a shape of their own, and then cuts it out and tapes it to the large sheet of paper. After that you can make contact.

EVALUATION:

In the follow-up discussion, discuss the two parts separately (the individual part and the part focused on contact):
- What does your own space look like?
- What is important about it, what colours does it have, what does the fence look like?
- Were you able to concentrate on yourself?
- Do you recognise this in connection with other situations?
- How did you want to make contact, and with whom?
- How did this go?
- What did you think of it, and is it recognisable or familiar to you?

10.14 ASSIGNMENT 12: Still Life Exercise: Asking and Refusing

Everyone chooses an object in the room (or chooses from a collection of objects) and together, the objects are used to create a still life on the table.

Then each client individually makes a pencil drawing in a rough outline of the still life as it has been placed on the table (no shading or hatching). The background is indicated by a few lines. Time: maximum of 10 minutes.

Then everyone takes a palette with paint in one colour and a fine brush. The therapist instructs: 'Now paint one part of your drawing in your own colour. After that, ask the others to paint one surface in your drawing, using their paint. Others will ask the same of you. In this way, you will gradually fill out your own work and each other's as well. There is also a catch: you must say no at least once. It's up to you when you say no and to whom'.

OBJECT:

Learning to ask for what you want.
Learning to say no.
Learning to combine different tasks.

MATERIALS:

Objects for a still life
Paper
Pencil
Paint in various colours
Fine brushes.

INDIVIDUAL/GROUP

EXPLANATORY NOTES:

In this assignment, no further arrangements are agreed, such as: don't all say no to the same person. Clients who are afraid of being rejected may discover that it won't be as bad as all that!
It may be a fairly confrontational manner of working because how things go is so clearly visible; for example, someone may forget about his own work, or may be the first one to finish.
Getting no as an answer can be very difficult and may evoke different reactions.

EVALUATION:

- Were you able to make sure that your own work was coloured completely? How did you ask the questions? What did others notice about this aspect?
- What was it like to say no? Was it easy or difficult? Did you think about which person you would say no to? Did everyone carry out this task?
- What was it like to get no for an answer? What was your reaction?

10.15 ASSIGNMENT 13: Clay Island

Place a large sheet of paper on the table so that when the group members stand around the table, they can reach everything (80–100 cm × 1.10 cm, approximately).

A large quantity of clay is ready and the group members are invited to take pieces of it and knead them. After kneading, the pieces of clay are thrown on the paper on the table, so that they become flat. The group continues to do this for a while (perhaps with noise from the material and their voices!), the idea being that the result will be a large island or island group.

When all the clay has been used, the group can develop the island by shaping it into mountains, plains, rocky coasts, rivers and lakes. Then the surroundings (the paper that is still visible) are painted using blue, white and green finger paint, so that a sea appears.

The island can be developed with all kinds of materials such as twigs, pebbles and so on (whatever is available). Now, everyone is asked to pick their own spot on the island and to fill in this spot to their liking. In the final step, everyone may make a small figure out of clay to represent themselves. This figure is given a place somewhere on the island.

OBJECT:

Learning to enjoy and savour life in a balanced manner.
Learning to play, shape and create something and work together.
Gaining insight into processes within the group.
Gaining insight into a shared interest versus individual needs.

MATERIALS:

A large sheet of paper, a large quantity of modelling clay (1 or 2 packs, depending on the size of the group), finger paints (blue, white, green), a variety of natural materials such as twigs, pebbles.

GROUP

EXPLANATORY NOTES:

The first phase is meant to loosen people up by letting them throw clay and make noise.

If the group is large, you could decide to work in subgroups so that there are several islands, resulting in comparison and competition.

EVALUATION:

- What was it like to do this assignment?
- How was your working relationship?
- What is important about or characteristic of the island?
- Does the island say something about how processes take place in the group, or about what group members think is important?
- Did a shared space emerge on the island, or a shared function?
- What does your own space look like? What was important when you were making it?
- Did everyone make figures and if so, where were they placed? What does the positioning tell you?

10.16 ASSIGNMENT 14: Black Lines, Group Assignment

Using a brush with black paint, all group members draw black lines on a large sheet.
After this, the black paint is put away and everyone chooses one colour of paint. Using this colour, everyone fills up the spaces between the black lines.

OBJECT:

Gaining insight into your own role or share in a cooperative project.
Becoming aware of what space you occupy.

MATERIALS:

School paint: black and various colours (as many colours as there are group members), brushes, a large sheet of paper on the table or the wall.

GROUP

EXPLANATORY NOTES:

This is a structured group assignment which in the first place is about jointly taking action, rather than a more individualised start. Later in the assignment, individual visibility in the group work will be a theme.

EVALUATION:

- Who took the initiative, who had a wait-and-see attitude?
- How carefully or how carelessly, or with how much freedom, did people work, and did you all agree on this? (group standard)
- How was your working relationship?
- What colour is the most predominant? What colour has the least space? What does this say about each group member's attitude and behaviour?
- Is this something you recognise from other group situations as well? (inside or outside the therapy programme)

10.17 ASSIGNMENT 15: Role-Playing with Instructions

Cards showing roles in the group are divided among the group members so that no one knows what role others were given (e.g. roles such as leader, protester, wait-and-see person, shy person, yes-man, clown, pusher, critic, carer, cooperative person, initiator).

The group is given a shared assignment with a fixed time limit:
- together, make a design for a holiday resort, a residential area or something similar
- together, paint a castle in natural surroundings
- make a building using drinking straws and tape
- make a structure using wine gums and wooden skewers
- make a structure from spaghetti
- etc.

OBJECT:

Becoming acquainted with group roles, learning to recognise and acknowledge your own group role.
Playing and practising with other group roles.

MATERIALS:

Depending on the assignment.

GROUP

EXPLANATORY NOTES:

The way a role is played says a great deal about the person playing it; in a leader role, a person can be authoritarian or democratic, for example. Often a person's previous experience, or how the person is accustomed to doing things, determines the direction.

If you carry out several short assignments in a row, you can let the group members choose their own role to practise in after the first round. As the therapist, you can also divide the roles on the basis of what is challenging for the group members, and suited to their treatment goals.

EVALUATION:

- What role did the group members think you had?
- What role did you have? How did you carry out this role? What was this like for others?
- What role do you play in other group situations?
- Do others recognise this as well?
- What would you like to practise or develop in this field?

10.18 ASSIGNMENT 16: Group Painting with Objectives

Decide what your treatment goals are in relation to social functioning (based on your treatment agreement or on experiences in previous sessions). Write them down.

Together, make a group painting on a large surface. While making a group painting, try to focus on your goals. Together, decide what the group painting will look like, whether other materials can be used as well and so on.

Optionally, halfway through the painting, there can be a moment of reflection during which all group members ask themselves whether they are still focused on their goals and how they want to continue working on them.

OBJECT:

Experimenting with and practising different behaviour, trying a different attitude in the group.
Gaining insight into social behaviour and into what you encounter when you change your own behaviour in the direction you have chosen.

MATERIALS:

Paint, a large sheet of paper: depending on group size.

GROUP

EXPLANATORY NOTES:

The group members must be somewhat familiar with each other, because this involves a great deal of interacting and working very closely together.

For this target group, working together is an activity that presents many difficulties and conflicts. This means that it can be a very tense or conflict-ridden assignment.

In the follow-up discussion, it is important to avoid being too judgemental ('it is not a good painting because people didn't work together') or discussing other people's attitudes rather than your own.

EVALUATION:

- What are your personal treatment goals in relation to social functioning?
- Which ones did you choose to practise in this assignment?
- How did it go?
- Did you stay focused on your goal or were you distracted from it?
- What did you see others doing differently than you are used to them doing?
- What did you think of this change?

10.19 ASSIGNMENT 17: Silhouettes. Group Task

On one wall, hang a very big sheet of paper in such a way that the tallest group member can still be drawn on it from head to toe, standing in front of it.

One at a time, a silhouette of each group member is made on this sheet of paper. Decide who you will choose to make your silhouette and give him or her the pencil. Stand against the sheet, choose a position and decide where and how you want to look. The person making the silhouette tries to follow the outline in as much detail as possible.

The person being drawn tries to focus on observing whether he or she feels physical tension and if so, where, and to what kind of behaviour or reaction he or she feels inclined in this situation.

Everyone gets a turn, while the rest of the group observes. Once all silhouettes are on the paper, the outlines are intensified by tracing over them with a colour or a black line. After this, everyone fills in his or her silhouette with paint in an abstract manner.

OBJECT:

Learning to occupy space, both literally and figuratively.
Feeling the tension created by having your silhouette drawn, where you feel this tension and what you do with it.
Becoming aware of and reflecting on your own issues in how you occupy space.

MATERIALS:

Very large sheet of paper (roll, 1.5 × 2.5 metres), pencil, school paint.

GROUP

EXPLANATORY NOTES:

Drawing each other's silhouette can be confrontational and can also be quite intimate.

In particular if it takes a long time, it can evoke a great deal of tension, certainly when the group is large and everyone is watching. And so it may be a good idea to intervene, depending on how much tension and/or light-heartedness is wanted.

An aspect of this expressive work worthy of attention is how group members deal with silhouettes that overlap: Who is part of the foreground, and who is part of the background, when the silhouettes are filled in later?

A variation on this is to work with a strong source of light (e.g. slide projector or overhead projector) so that there is more distance between the person being drawn and the person drawing the silhouette.

For a more harmonious or aesthetic final result, you could choose to work only in black and white or in one particular colour combination, for example.

EVALUATION:

- What was it like, having your outline drawn in pencil?
- Did this create tension in you, and how did you deal with this?
- What was your first reaction on seeing your own silhouette? Did you have an opinion about it, and if so, what did you think? Could you accept it as it was, or did you change something about it?
- How did you fill it in? Did you mean to show something by doing this?
- What did you do when silhouettes overlapped? Who became part of the foreground, who part of the background?
- What do all of you think of the end result?

10.20 ASSIGNMENT 18: Matisse Brushes

The therapist has prepared a wall or a floor (without the group having seen this) with a very big sheet of paper, and underneath it a smaller sheet, and under that an even smaller sheet (25 × 40 cm, for example).

Each group member chooses a colour of paint and puts a large quantity of it on a palette.

Then the Matisse bamboo sticks (large bamboo poles with brushes taped to the end) are taken out.

Everyone will paint on the large paper with the large brush until they all decide (in a non-verbal manner) that it is finished. While working, no one may speak.

Nothing further is agreed about what is to be painted, only that the sheet of paper must be covered completely (no white paper is visible) and that the painting is abstract. When it is finished, the paper is removed and put somewhere else. The slightly smaller sheet of paper is now visible, and the group continues its painting on that. After that, this sheet of paper is also removed, and the smallest sheet is painted completely full, until the group decides that it is finished.

OBJECT:

Learning to cooperate in situations with reduced control.
Learning to play.
Learning to handle conflicts.
Learning to retain the contact or the conflict as the space becomes smaller (and so everything comes closer).

MATERIALS:

Long bamboo poles (1.5 metres) with thick, round brushes taped to the ends, sheets of paper of approximately 2 × 2.5 metres, 1 × 1.20 metres and 0.30 × 0.40 metres, school paint (as many colours as there are group members).

GROUP

EXPLANATORY NOTES:

The surprise effect of the long brushes, the appearance of the smaller sheets of paper, all this is important for the pleasure taken in this assignment or the tension it arouses.

The long brushes make it much more difficult to paint with any control. The brushes bump into each other, your brush goes over someone else's work and so on. This makes a good exercise for a group in which the members are too cautious towards each other and for clients who are strongly focused on control. It increases spontaneity and as well as coincidences and surprises.

Optionally, this assignment can be done in pairs (e.g. in partner or relationship therapy as well) or in subgroups working with a single pole. Which roles are adopted (leading, following)? How do you work together?

EVALUATION:

- What was it like to work with the big brushes? Could you accept the fact that you had less control than you would normally have?
- How was your working relationship?
- What was it like to work with each other on a territory that became smaller and smaller?
- What effect did the shrinking format have; did tension rise, was there more conflict about space, was there more intimacy?
- Did you have to forgo something on account of the smaller format?
- Did everyone go on painting or did some people stop; did they shy away from contact?

10.21 ASSIGNMENT 19: Boat with Crew

Together with the group, paint a large boat. Don't discuss it beforehand, just go ahead and paint.
In the last 10 minutes, each group member will paint himself or herself somewhere on the boat. Each of you should think about where and how you would like to see yourself on the boat, or perhaps what your function is on the boat, and then just go ahead and paint yourself without any consultation.

OBJECT:

Becoming aware of and discussing the various roles and positions in the group.
Taking a stand on your ideas about your own position.
Becoming aware of reactions to positions people have.

MATERIALS:

Large format paper (1 × 2 metres), school paint, brushes.

GROUP

EXPLANATORY NOTES:

This assignment is also useful if a crisis occurs in the group. It makes the positions clear.

EVALUATION:

- How was your working relationship in making the boat?
- Who took the initiative, who looked after the things, who decided what the boat would be like?
- Where and how did you put yourself on the boat, what was your function?
- How do others see this?
- Does this correspond to the attitude you adopted when working together on this assignment?
- If not, why not?

10.22 ASSIGNMENT 20: Tower Made from Newspapers, with Handicap

Divide the group into two smaller groups of equal size (at least 3 persons per group). The idea is that each group uses newspapers, tape and/or string to build a freestanding tower that is as high as possible.

Before starting, the groups devise a handicap for each member of the other group. The handicaps are then applied on each person. Examples of handicaps are immobilising body parts by taping them or blindfolding people. If a person is very unhappy with a particular handicap, it may be refused, and the group will devise another one. Once everyone has a handicap, they can start.

The therapist keeps track of the time, for example, half an hour. The object is to make the highest or the best-looking tower.

OBJECT:

Learning to work together.
Allowing yourself to be playful about competing and challenging others.

MATERIALS:

Stacks of newspapers, 1 roll of tape, 1 pair of scissors and string for each group.

GROUP

EXPLANATORY NOTES:

Because the two small groups work alongside each other, this immediately brings competition, excitement and fun.

Actually working together is more difficult on account of the handicaps, which can make things quite awkward. A point to be observed is how people react to their own handicap—for example, does a person become very passive and withdraw if he or she cannot see anything? How do they react to the handicaps of others? What can another person still do despite the handicap, and how do the other group members respond to this? Each group is given only one roll of tape and 1 pair of scissors, which means they will need each other in order to work together.

EVALUATION:

- What was it like to devise handicaps for the other group?
- How did you work together in your own group?
- How did you deal with your own handicap while working?
- How did you deal with handicaps of other group members that limited how much they could do?
- Do you recognise yourself in this in how you work together with others in different situations?
- Was it important to win? How enthusiastic or fanatical were you?

10.23 ASSIGNMENT 21: A Drawing Dialogue

Hang up a sheet of paper, or fasten it to the table. The group sits down around it. Everyone chooses 2 or 3 colours of chalk.

One person starts drawing and continues to draw until he or she has had enough, and stops. This is the signal that another group member must take the initiative and continue drawing on the sheet of paper. This person continues drawing until he or she decides to stop. Now, someone else takes over. The idea is not to draw in a certain order; a person may have more than one turn, and the time that a person works on the drawing may vary greatly (sometimes briefly, sometimes a bit longer).

OBJECT:

Learning to take up space, to have a presence.
Coordinating your work with others.
Taking initiatives.
Being able to stop and allow another person some space.

MATERIALS:

For pairs: a sheet of paper of 80 × 100 cm.
For a group: A sheet of paper of 1 × 1.50 metres, or according to group size.
Pastels or oil pastels.

PAIRS/GROUP

EXPLANATORY NOTES:

This assignment can be done in pairs or in two subgroups. The latter yields more interaction. In a larger group, it may be more stressful to take the initiative.

A variation on this assignment is that your turn ends when a group member puts his or her chalk on the paper. This is the signal for the person drawing that it is time to stop. It yields a different dynamic than waiting until the person drawing decides to stop. Things sometimes become more playful when another person's turn can be appropriated; there may be more room for trying out things like teasing and working very rapidly. In such cases, you have to seize your turn; it is not given to you. Which form is the most suitable depends on the size of the group. It is also conceivable that both variations are used one after the other, so that the group can discuss the differences they perceived.

EVALUATION:

- What was it like to do this assignment?
- Were you able to seize your turn?
- Were you able to take the initiative?
- Did you primarily draw new ideas, or your own ideas, or did you add to what was already on the paper?
- What title would you give the drawing, or the dialogue?
- What is characteristic of the dialogue that took place? Is this familiar to you?

11

Distress Tolerance Skills Module

11.1 Summary of Distress Tolerance Skills Theory

Dialectical behaviour therapy emphasises bearing pain skilfully. For our mental health, the capacity to bear and to accept distress is of great importance for the two following reasons.

Pain and crises are part of life, they cannot be avoided or eliminated completely. Inability to accept this fact only leads to more pain and suffering.

Bearing crises, at least in the short term, is an essential part of every attempt to change yourself; otherwise, impulsive acts will undermine attempts to achieve the desired changes.

The object is to accept the crisis situation as it is, in a non-evaluative and non-judgemental manner. This is the capacity to observe your surroundings without asking them to change, to experience your present emotional state without trying to change it and to observe behavioural patterns without trying to stop them or control them. It is very important to realise that accepting reality is not the same thing as condoning it!

S. Haeyen, *Art Therapy and Emotion Regulation Problems*,
https://doi.org/10.1007/978-3-319-96773-8_11

Two skills are taught in this module:

- Learning to accept life as it is now.
- Learning to accept a crisis and live through it.

Accepting Life as It Is Now

Accepting reality means learning acceptance skills and willingness instead of being stubborn. Avoiding everything that has to do with pain simply means the pain continues to exist. Attempts to suppress emotional pain or to avoid everything that is painful lead to worrying about the painful events. This means it is important that a person chooses to accept the pain. This means full acceptance, an active inner process to learn to accept reality as it is. Willingness means declaring that you are ready to take part: saying yes. Stubbornness is staying on the sidelines in an attempt to control the course of events: saying no, or yes, but.

Accepting and Living Through a Crisis

The strategies for accepting and living through a crisis are learned in four groups of skills: distraction, cherishing yourself, improving the moment and focusing attention on advantages and disadvantages.

Experiencing emotional pain, enduring and accepting it are the ways in which pain is reduced. Sometimes a situation is too difficult or too painful to be processed immediately, and in that case, it is better to seek temporary distraction. Then it is important to make measured contact with your emotions.

The skills in this module are in fact ways of surviving and doing what is right in unpleasant situations without turning to conduct that would only compound them. The basic idea is how to get through unpleasant situations without making matters worse.

In this module, we will look at the pan scale, a scale that charts five degrees of mounting tension for identifying and influencing crises. There is attention to the moment in the form of awareness and relaxation exercises. If these exercises are done every day, they can help clients develop a state of mind more open to acceptance. Clients will learn to look closely at pain and to analyse the crisis situation.

11.2 Multidisciplinary Relationships in the Various Aspects of Treatment

Dialectical behaviour therapy, module: distress tolerance skills
Pain and crisis are part of life. Inability to accept this fact leads to more pain and suffering

Distress tolerance skills: Skills for accepting and living through a crisis. Accepting life as it is now (accepting reality)

Skills training	Psycho-education: a crisis situation must be endured in a non-evaluative and non-judgemental manner Drawing up a crisis identification plan, practising willingness and acceptance
Homework	Working method: Complete the crisis identification plan
Basic group	Unstructured group in which, for example, members can discuss their experiences with crisis situations
Art therapy	Making helpful symbols that can be supportive in a crisis—for example, something that symbolises a characteristic or skill, such as a soapstone that you can take with you, a reminder card or a figure. This makes their help real, concrete and tangible and so it will be present outside the therapy for transfer purposes Portraying the 'five pans' scale Actively seeking pleasant situations, safety and distraction in shaping and experiencing the materials (nurturing your senses). Giving shape to a safe place, perhaps an imaginary one. Finding ways to work in art therapy that provide pleasant distraction
Music therapy	Attention to interaction with music at home. What music helps you to relax, release tension, be able to cry. What music makes you aggressive or sombre. Getting the do's and don'ts straight. Actively learning to stop playing or turn interaction in a different direction Composing your own rap, for example, and looking for other ways to make room for acute tension and emotions in a healthy manner. A homework assignment to investigate what is realistic

Psychomotor therapy	Learning to recognise body signals that are part of a crisis Experiencing crisis situations (with your eyes closed, higher up) and finding ways to deal with it (such as doing breathing exercises, asking for help) Relaxation or breathing exercises, discovering what types of movement can bring distraction. Attention to others (e.g. as a group, make a chair for the other person), attention-focusing exercises (such as running)
Sociotherapy starting and ending the daily session/ environment	Looking into what you need if tension at home runs high: when will you look for distraction, when will you contact a friend, when will you ask for a timeout, make plans

11.3 ASSIGNMENT 1: Clay in a Bag

Step 1:
'Everyone takes a plastic bag in a dark colour in which they can easily move their hands. Everyone takes a piece of clay, not too small, but what feels comfortable in your hand. Everyone takes the clay in their hands, and puts their hands into the plastic bag. Concentrate on feeling your way and without being able to see what you are doing, make a ball from the clay. There is no talking during this exercise; just concentrate on yourself'.

Step 2:
After about five minutes, everyone stops work on making a ball. 'Take a minute to observe and feel the ball and then you and the person sitting next to you exchange clay balls. Now, observe how different the other person's ball feels (temperature, moisture, smoothness, form and weight). Talk about it with your neighbour, and then exchange clay balls again'.

Step 3:
'You have your own bag with the clay ball. Now, you can knead the clay some more and follow what your hands want to do. In this manner, a shape will be produced; it may be something recognisable, but not necessarily so. No peeking into the bag when the exercise is over!' (See evaluation.)

OBJECT:

Observing using your sense of touch, enjoying this.
Learning to focus your attention and to concentrate on the here and now.
Learning to accept the result that arises in this situation with reduced control.

MATERIALS:

Clay, black plastic bags (large enough to work in with both hands and the clay).

INDIVIDUALLY in the Group

EXPLANATORY NOTES:

Variation: In step 3, choose a theme if you want to work with more structure or direction.
If a feeling is apparent in the group—for example, dissatisfaction—this could be used as a theme. If you or the group prefer a more specific assignment, make an animal or an object.
If a person might decompensate, this exercise is counter-indicated.

EVALUATION:

At the beginning of the follow-up discussion, you may not look inside the bag.

- What has the clay inside the bag turned into? What does it look like and (what skills and how skills) how did the process take place?

After these discussion points, the clay is removed from the bag.
- Is the image you had in mind different to the actual clay object?

(It is worthy of note that the image in a person's mind and the way it actually looks can be perceived very differently.) Ask everyone to put this experience into words. What often happens is that at first, people talk about the experience quite non-judgementally but as soon as they have had a look, they do judge and even reject the product. It is important to be aware of this because it is something that probably takes place quite often: the actual experience goes smoothly but later, people are judgemental and the entire experience is thus devalued.

11.4 ASSIGNMENT 2: Problems and Solutions

The therapist instructs:
'In the middle of the paper, make a circle and divide the rest of the paper into a number of boxes, as many as there are group members present, by drawing lines from the circle to the edge of the paper'.
'In the circle, make a picture of a difficult situation, something you have run into that you have trouble with, by for example symbolising it on the paper (10 minutes). After that, we will go around the table briefly so that everyone can explain what they drew and what problem it represents'.
'Now pass the paper to the person on your left. In one of the boxes, this person may react to the problem in the circle by naming an imaginary suggestion or a solution to the problem. Then pass the paper to the next person on the left, until all the boxes have been filled in'.
(Be sure to divide the time so that all group members have a turn).
'If a solution to a problem has already been represented, the person whose turn it is must try to devise something else instead. So do your best to think up a creative solution, perhaps something quite different!'

Finally, the paper comes back to the person who filled the circle in the middle, with all the reactions of the group members on it.

OBJECT:

Being able to empathise with one another.
Receiving help and new ideas from group members.
Receiving other points of view or different perspectives to your problem.
Increasing your problem-solving capacity, thinking divergently.

MATERIALS:

Paper (at least A3) and crayons.

GROUP

EXPLANATORY NOTES:

This exercise can also be carried out individually if desired. In that case, the person who has presented the difficult situation must seek several solutions and picture them. This can help people learn to think in more than one direction for a solution.

EVALUATION:

Group members can explain their suggestions, reactions and/or solutions. Go around the table for each work. Then ask a few questions of the person whose work it is.

- Which of the solutions would be a good option for you?
- Which of the solutions provides you with a new or unexpected perspective?
- How does it feel to be given these suggestions, reactions and solutions?

11.5 ASSIGNMENT 3: Giving and Receiving Feedback

1. 'From the picture collection of men and women, each group member chooses pictures for each other group member, pictures that they think would suit him or her, because of who he or she is or because this is what you would wish for them' (from the pictures file, see Annex 2).

'Probably the most obvious thing to do is to choose pictures of men for the men and pictures of women for the women, but you may decide to do this differently. Lastly, choose one picture for yourself'.
2. The pictures are given to the group members, but without any explanation at this point.
3. Going around the group briefly, everyone responds to the pictures they received and explains the picture they chose for themselves. After this, the group members who gave pictures may explain why they made this choice. In this exercise, the primary focus is differences in interpretation between the recipient of the feedback and the person who gave it.
4. 'Based on the pictures and the feedback received, make an expressive work using materials and techniques of your choice. It is completely up to you what you want to work on, whatever is important to you'.

Note: The order in which parts 3 and 4 are carried out can be reversed, so that first an expressive work is made, followed by explanations or information.

OBJECT:

Working together.
Giving and receiving feedback.
Gaining insight into how your own interpretation can change.
Conflict management.

MATERIALS:

Pictures file: categories of men and women, free choice of materials for the expressive work.

GROUP

EXPLANATORY NOTES:

Reversing the order of parts 3 and 4 yields a bigger surprise effect, but whether this is a good idea depends on the target group. It can make the exercise more confrontational.
If the initial order is used, clients can more readily decide what they want to keep for themselves, or what they want to work on. It gives them greater control, making it more suitable for people with less ego strength.

EVALUATION:

- What is it like to give feedback; what sort of tension does this evoke?
- What is it like to receive feedback?
- Are you able to give feedback that may be confrontational, or do you prefer to keep everything positive, or formulated in the form of wishes?
- Is there a difference between how someone else intended the picture and how you took it; what does this say about you? (And about the person who gave it?)
- Linking this to daily life: do you recognise these aspects in how you normally deal with things?
- What did you decide to make in the expressive work?
- What did you make, and how did you do this?
- Is there a link between the manner in which you worked expressively and the feedback?

11.6 ASSIGNMENT 4: Positive Book (Follow-Up to Assignment on Giving and Receiving Feedback)

The therapist instructs:
'Using copies of the pictures from assignment 3 (giving and receiving feedback), make a book in which you present a collection of all kinds of things that make you feel good and that can offer support in a crisis situation.

- pictures of people, animals or situations that are dear to you
- pictures, texts and symbols
- helpful thoughts
- pleasant activities and places

You have two sessions in which to complete this'.

Homework:
'Ask at least three (!) people in your surroundings for positive feedback. Ask them to write this down, and ask if they might want to include a suitable picture. Bring this with you next time to use in making the positive book'.

OBJECT:

In moments of crisis or when you are sombre, being able to fall back on and hold on to positive feelings about yourself or others.
Holding on to positive experiences and memories.
Learning to provide support for yourself.
Learning to keep on focusing, on positive things as well.

MATERIALS:

Coloured paper, newspapers, materials to bind the book, string.
Photographs and letters brought by the client.
Perhaps a laminator with which to make a sturdy book cover.
Hole punch, stapler.

INDIVIDUALLY in the Group

EXPLANATORY NOTES:

The target group is accustomed to focus totally on negative aspects in moments of sombreness and crisis and to allow themselves to be carried away by the feeling of the moment. This exercise emphasises holding on to a reality that has both positive and negative aspects.
Asking people you are close to for feedback is something that people are not used to doing, but it has great effect and often adds value. This thought helps people to get over the threshold (to ask for feedback); people often find it difficult or awkward to ask for it.

EVALUATION:

For the evaluation, the person who made the book is asked to present it.

- What was it like to ask for and receive feedback, from your own surroundings as well?
- Would you like to show something of it, or read some of it to us?
- What did it do with you, making this collection?
- Is it something you will really be able to use in difficult moments?

11.7 ASSIGNMENT 5: Helpful Symbol

1. Paint or draw yourself in a situation that you find difficult (10 minutes). Brief interim discussion: What situation did you represent? What sort of feeling does it give you?
2. Think about a skill or characteristic that could help you in this situation. Make a symbol for this (25 minutes).
3. Make the symbol on a sticky label as well and stick it on a place where you will see it regularly (your diary, a mirror, in your purse) as a reminder of the skill or characteristic that you want to develop. You can also put it on a small card (about the size of your bank card) and laminate it. Then you can easily put it in your purse.

OBJECT:

Counteracting and correcting dysfunctional behaviour, emotions, thoughts.
Focusing on and confirming the skill or characteristic the client wants to develop.
Turning this into a helpful symbol that will serve as a reminder.

MATERIALS:

Drawing and painting materials, sticky labels, cards, laminator and laminating pouches.

INDIVIDUALLY in the Group

EXPLANATORY NOTES:

A helpful symbol can be useful in many situations, such as a reminder of how to reduce tension rather than allow it to build up (see the pan scale).

EVALUATION:

- What did you make to use as a symbol and what does it stand for?
- Where are you planning to put the sticker, or keep or put the card?
- Will you see it there often enough?

Optionally, come back to this in the next session:

- Where is the sticker/the card, and have you looked at it, was it helpful to you?

11.8 ASSIGNMENT 6: Pleasant Spot, 3D

The therapist instructs:
'Make a base with an upright wall at the back out of sturdy carton with the help of two triangular side walls. This forms a backdrop where you can design your own space. It is your personal space. It does not need to be a place that actually exists. First paint it, affix stickers to it or make it look nice, and then add whatever else you want.
What sort of atmosphere do you want this spot to have? What would you enjoy finding in it? Would you want one or several doors or shutters in the side walls or the back wall?
Make whatever you think belongs there, whatever you need'.

OBJECT:

Focusing on and becoming aware of your own sense of safety. (how is this feeling created, what do you need?)

MATERIALS:

Greyboard, coloured paper, paints, strong tape.
Bits of fabric, wool, feathers, junk, natural materials such as sand, pebbles, leaves.

INDIVIDUALLY in the Group

EXPLANATORY NOTES:

The doors or shutters can offer an opportunity for relaxation and may also give onto other spots (e.g. an anxious, unpleasant place) that you might decide to build onto your personal space. Doing this assignment will require several sessions.

EVALUATION:

- What was it like to work on this place of your own?
- How did you design and furnish this spot (colour, design elements, atmosphere)?
- What makes this spot pleasant or safe?
- What do you need from this place, what is important about it?
- Are there doors or shutters in the side walls or the back wall? What is their function?

11.9 ASSIGNMENT 7: Pans

The pan scale is an emotional intensity scale in 5 steps (with 5 pans) as used in the Dutch VERS training, comparable to STEPPS, a emotion and behaviour management skills training (Harvey, Blum, Black, Burgess, & Henley-Cragg, 2014).
The pan scale goes from pan 1 (the water in the pan is calm): complete relaxation, to pan 5 (the pan is boiling over): complete emotional outburst. Using the pan scale, clients chart their increasing tension and learn how to recognise their tension level, how they can prevent any further increase and how they may be able to reduce their tension level by adjusting their behaviour.

The therapist instructs:
'Determine how the pans look (in pictures) when applied to your experience of how tension rises in you (and what you then feel, think and do).
Make five different pictures (in a single work or in five separate parts) showing the various pans. Use shapes, colours, images, text and materials. You might also try to adjust the way in which you work with the materials

to the pan you are picturing. For example, working with chalk in pan 1 gives a soft and even surface. Pan 5 will probably be brightly coloured and full of scratches'.
Two sessions are needed for this assignment.

OBJECT:

Distinguishing and classifying the various tension levels.
Gaining insight into how tension builds up in you.
Learning to fine-tune between the various tension levels.
Gaining insight into your influence on how tension builds in you, how to stabilise it and how to reduce it.

MATERIALS:

Free choice.

INDIVIDUALLY

EXPLANATORY NOTES:

It may be difficult to distinguish five different levels in the way your tension can build. It is advisable to start with pans that are easy to recognise: pan 1 and pan 5. This can vary greatly from one person to another; some clients do not have pan 1 (they always have some tension, so pan 2) and others have no pan 5 (they never lose control completely).

It can be interesting if making a picture on the basis of a tension level appropriate to pan 4 or 5 is found to be agreeable. When tension peaks, it can also be regarded as a moment of strength, of spontaneity. From this point of view, tension build-up can be seen as not only a destructive pattern, but also as something constructive.

After this, clients may choose to work out one pan in more detail or to try using some different materials, experimenting with or practising different behaviour in making expressive works.

EVALUATION:

- What was it like to do this assignment?
- Were some of the pans more difficult and others easier to draw?
- Does your way of working with the material connect to the tension level in the pan?
- What do you do that causes tension to build so that you find yourself in the next pan?
- What can you do to prevent this, to stabilise or reduce the tension?
- What pan are you in right now?

11.10 ASSIGNMENT 8: Treasuring Something Beautiful

Before doing this assignment, ask clients to bring a picture that they think is beautiful. It may be something that already has a place of its own at home, a picture that someone has kept for a while or a picture that someone decides to find for this occasion.
Ask clients to choose a detail or a part of it to work on. Make sure that people do not set to work in a perfectionist manner. It may be helpful to work from two-dimensional to three-dimensional (or vice versa) so that what a client makes is not a reproduction, but transposes the picture into the client's own personal design. This can also strengthen the sensory experience.

OBJECT:

Treasuring pleasant images.
Attending to the senses, treasuring them.
Focusing on the moment.

MATERIALS:

Free choice.

INDIVIDUALLY

EXPLANATORY NOTES:

The use of materials such as small bits of soapstone, clay, fabrics and similar materials is advised to stimulate sensory perception, particularly touch.

EVALUATION:

- What picture was your starting point and why did you choose it?
- What aspect or what part of it did you choose to work out in your own way?
- What was it like to do this?
- Were you able to make your own transposition of the picture?
- What materials did you use, and what did it feel like to work with them?
- What would you like to do with the finished product? Would you like to put it on a table, lay it down or hang it up in your home?

11.11 ASSIGNMENT 9: Holiday from Adulthood

Working on the basis of the above theme, clients (as a group, in pairs or individually) make a messy painting using finger paint or school paint. There are no further rules or working arrangements, only the theme.

OBJECT:

Relaxing, letting go of demands or expectations.
Observing non-judgementally.
Participating.

MATERIALS:

Sponge, brushes, paper (from a roll), large format.

GROUP/IN PAIRS/INDIVIDUALLY

EXPLANATORY NOTES:

This can be done either in the group or individually. The main object is enjoying yourself; it does not need to mean anything or represent anything.

EVALUATION:

- What was it like to do this?

The follow-up discussion should not last too long and certainly not be too serious. It is the experience itself that is important, and not thoughts or opinions.

11.12 ASSIGNMENT 10: Dream Holiday

The therapist instructs:
'Make a picture of your dream holiday. Everything is allowed. You can go where you want; there are no restrictions. You can take everyone along or leave them all home. Where would you go? What simply must be there? Try to put across the atmosphere you have in mind as well as possible with the picture'.

This assignment can be done individually, in pairs or as a group assignment.
The most important thing is that the picture is developed to represent a fantasy of the most ideal holiday without any restrictions based on reality.

OBJECT:

Enjoying the moment.
Relaxing.
Treasuring a pleasant feeling.

MATERIALS:

Collage, paint or crayons, or free choice.

GROUP/IN PAIRS/INDIVIDUALLY

EXPLANATORY NOTES:

If they like, clients can also make a postcard they will send home. On the front, it will show a picture of the holiday (a pretend photo) and on the back a text, the addressee and the sender.

EVALUATION:

- What does your dream holiday look like?
- What is so nice or pleasant about it?

It is recommended to keep the evaluation brief. The experience should not be talked to death. For example, stay in the fantasy of the dream holiday:

- What does a day of your holiday look like: Where are you, what do you do? How do you feel there?
- Who is there with you? Are you by yourself?
- What would you write on a postcard to send home?

11.13 ASSIGNMENT 11: Senses—Sensations

Part 1: Seek out a material with which you express two contrasting sensations (hard–soft, wet–dry, bright–pastel). Investigate which contrast you want to use and in what way you can show it the most strongly. In doing so, think of your various senses; for instance, you can focus on what you see, on what you feel, on what you hear.

Part 2: Work out the contrasting sensations on the basis of what gives you a pleasant or good feeling.

OBJECT:

Investigating, recognising and acknowledging your own perceptions and needs.
Observing sensory experiences.
Being able to give shape to and describe your own perception and or your own needs.

MATERIALS:

Variety of materials.

GROUP/IN PAIRS/INDIVIDUALLY

EXPLANATORY NOTES:

This can be done either individually or together with others (which will involve aspects of cooperation).

EVALUATION:

- What contrast did you investigate with the material? What did the two opposites arouse in you?
- What did you observe through your senses?
- What manner of working gave you a good or pleasant feeling? Describe it.
- What was it like to continue working on this?
- Do you often have this feeling in your daily life, and what do you do with it then? Would you like to have this feeling more often, and how can you make sure you do? Is this advisable, a good idea?

11.14 ASSIGNMENT 12: Meditation Image

Clients make a shape that is appropriate to equilibrium, harmony/being non-judgemental and accepting. Optionally, this assignment can be introduced with a guided fantasy.

A mandala can also be a more structured interpretation of this assignment for clients who have a hard time thinking up something on their own. In that case, everyone makes their own mandala, a circle that is filled in with contrasting shapes and colours. Clients may also choose to work with a compass and examples of mandalas.

OBJECT:

Focusing on balance and harmony.
Working with acceptance and structure.

MATERIALS:

Free choice, for the mandala: paper, compass, pencil or coloured pencils, paint.

INDIVIDUALLY in the Group

EXPLANATORY NOTES:

The personal meditation figure can be taken home so that it can be used as a support to help clients focus on balance, harmony and acceptance.

EVALUATION:

- How did you work on this?
- Did you immediately know what you wanted to make?
- Is it an existing image or a new image for you?
- What does this image mean to you?
- Where will you put it if you take it home? Can you imagine that you use the image to look at very purposely for a few minutes every day and to meditate?

Next time, ask where they put the mandala and whether it helped them to reflect on balance and acceptance.

11.15 ASSIGNMENT 13: Copying a Painting

The therapist instructs:
'Choose an abstract painting in an art book and copy the painting (or part of it) as closely as you can. If you like, you can add something to it or change it to suit your own insights'.

OBJECT:

Seeking distraction.
Concentrating on something outside yourself.

MATERIALS:

Paint, paper, art books, pictures of paintings.

GROUP/IN PAIRS/INDIVIDUALLY

EXPLANATORY NOTES:

This assignment can also be carried out in pairs.
The manner of painting used in the picture can be quite different to what the client is used to. This means it can be a new experience, in which clients practise and experience a different manner of working.

Variation: enlarge or zoom in on a part of the painting and copy this part. If clients want to copy the painting exactly, a drawback can be that they become focused on precision and perfectionism. For this reason, work with time limits or with wide brushes as interventions to counter this tendency. Stress the fact that the idea is not to make an exact copy.

EVALUATION:

- How did you come to choose this painting?
- What was it like to copy this painting, or part of it?
- Were you able to concentrate?
- Were you able to find distraction in working on it? (Perhaps you can link this to the client's mood on arrival.)
- What manner of painting is used in the example, and what was it like to try to do this as well? How did you experience this? Is this an entirely different manner to what you are used to? Would you like to work in this way more often?

11.16 ASSIGNMENT 14: Secret Room in Yourself

The therapist instructs:
'Imagine a secret room in yourself and see what it looks like. It is a room in which you relax, to which you retreat when you feel endangered or

threatened. The door is closed to everything that might hurt you. The room is calming, pleasant and lovely'.

The following text can serve as a source of inspiration:

I have a house where I go
When there's too many people,
I have a house where I go
Where no one can be;
I have a house where I go
Where nobody ever says "No";
Where no one says anything–so
There is no one but me.

(Reference: A.A. Milne, *Now We Are Six*, Copyright, 1927, by E.P. Dutton & Co., Inc., Copyright Renewal, 1955, by A.A. Milne, p. 131.)

OBJECT:

Finding peace and quiet for yourself.
Looking for safety in yourself and giving it tangible shape.

MATERIALS:

Free choice.

INDIVIDUALLY

EXPLANATORY NOTES:

The secret room is used here as a symbol for the safety inside yourself. By making it more tangible, it may be easier to actively seek out this feeling, to experience it and hold on to it.

EVALUATION:

- Would you show us your secret room and tell us something about it? It's up to you; after all, it's your private property (actively offer a choice).

If so:

- How did you design your secret room; what was important in it? What makes it safe?
- Do you need this room often? Has this always been the same, or was there a time when you needed it more?
- In your daily life, is there a place in your surroundings where you can feel like this? And do you use it?
- The portrayal you made of your secret room, have you had that idea for some time?

11.17 ASSIGNMENT 15: Something Nice for Someone Else

The therapist instructs:
'Make something nice, something personal for the person on your right (symbolic gifts). What do you think that person needs? What would make him or her happy?'

OBJECT:

Paying attention to others.
Giving and receiving positive feedback.

MATERIALS:

Free choice.

INDIVIDUALLY in the Group

EXPLANATORY NOTES:

In a crisis situation, people often pay disproportionate attention to themselves. In such a case, seeking distraction and focusing attention on another person are a learning point.

Variation: Make something nice, a gift for yourself. This variation can be used when a person has little positive attention to himself or herself (low self-esteem, little self-care) and focuses too much on others.

EVALUATION:

- Were you able to focus your attention on the other person?
- Could you be sensitive, understanding, to him or her? (can also be estimated based on the reaction of the other person)
- What do you think of the gift you were given?
- Do you recognise the gift made for you as something you were in need of?
- Do you have the feeling that the other person empathised with you?

11.18 ASSIGNMENT 16: Pain

The therapist instructs:
'In your thoughts, go to the theme of emotional pain.
When did you feel this kind of pain, and what did it have to do with? Where did you feel pain? Did you also have physical reactions? What does it do to you if you think about that pain again right now? How could you give shape to that pain, a pain that may recur when you hear these questions?

Make a personal portrayal of the theme of pain. Do this symbolically (figuratively or in the abstract) or purely material-based by using the materials in a certain way. You may also combine several materials'.

OBJECT:

Acknowledging pain instead of avoiding it.
Exploring, recognising and acknowledging your own emotional pain.

MATERIALS:

Free choice.

INDIVIDUALLY in the Group

EXPLANATORY NOTES:

Avoiding everything that has to do with pain allows the pain to continue to exist. Attempts to suppress emotional pain or to avoid everything that is painful lead to worrying about the painful events.

Follow-up assignment/part 2: **Seal off the pain**
(you may want to do this in the next session in order to give it enough attention).
In your work that reflects or symbolises the pain, make something that seals off the pain.

OBJECT:

- Learning to define limits for pain.
- Separating yourself from pain.

EVALUATION:

In the evaluation, do not go into the depth on the emotional pain or experiences related to it. The focus is how people deal with it.

- What did you make?
- Describe your work in terms of what skills and how skills.
- How did you handle the theme of emotional pain: in the materials you used, in what you do when you start to feel it?
- What significance does the work have for you, and what is it like to look at it?

11.19 ASSIGNMENT 17: Be Proud of Yourself!

Start with either exercise 1 or 2.

Part 1.
'On a sheet of paper, write a list with 10 qualities that you have. They may be skills or characteristics, things that you know belong with your character, or things that you have learned. They may be things that are mainly important for you as an individual, or perhaps things that come forward precisely in contact with others'.
(You may also assign the written part of this first exercise as homework in the preceding session. In that case, clients could ask a few people in their immediate environs to make some additions to the list.)
'Stand in a circle as a group, holding your list in your hand. Walk to one person at a time in the circle and say to that person: "I am ... and my qualities are ..."'.
Brief follow-up discussion about the question: Was it stressful, and were you able to handle the tension? How?

Part 2.
(Optionally, with a brief imagination exercise) 'Think back to a situation, not long ago, in which you were proud of yourself or satisfied with the way you acted. Make an expressive work showing the feeling of pride or showing the situation it involved'.

OBJECT:

Learning to remember better times when a crisis occurs.
Being able to hold on to a positive experience.
Self-empowerment: becoming aware of your own qualities. Discovering, recognising, acknowledging.
Allowing yourself to experience pride, ego reinforcement, increasing self-confidence.

MATERIALS:

Free choice.

INDIVIDUALLY in the Group

EXPLANATORY NOTES:

Referring to the individual treatment goals may help people seek out a situation about which they feel satisfaction.

EVALUATION:

- What situation did you choose, and why?
- What were you proud of?
- What is it like to look at this work now?
- Are you often proud of yourself, or only once in a while? Is this realistic?

11.20 ASSIGNMENT 18: The Leaf

The therapist instructs:
'Sit down, relaxed, in your chair with your arms on the arm rests, your feet slightly apart directly under your knees, pointing straight ahead. You may close your eyes if you wish. If you prefer not to, then look at a still spot in the room – for example, at the floor in front of you. Try to relax the muscles in your face, your neck, your chest, your abdomen, your arms and legs. The follow your breathing as it enters your body, goes to your abdomen, and comes slowly back out. Follow your breathing once more, from outside to inside and back out again.
Imagine that you are a leaf hanging on the branch of a tree in a forest. A light breeze blows you off the branch. Slowly, you flutter to the ground. This trip takes you past many other leaves and branches. You follow the trunk of the tree and you land gently on a murmuring brook flowing through the forest. You are surrounded by the cool water, and very slowly, you flutter towards the bottom of the water. You feel very light; borne by the water, you slowly sink deeper and deeper, until you cautiously land on the bottom of the brook. The leaf settles there quietly.
Now, follow your breathing as it enters your body, goes to your abdomen, and slowly comes back out. Follow your breathing once more, from outside to inside and back out again. Prepare yourself to come back into the

room. Follow your breathing twice more, from outside to inside and back again, and then open your eyes. You may feel rested and refreshed'.

'Take the feeling you had during this exercise as the starting point for an expressive work. Choose materials that you think are appropriate to this. While working, try to hold on to this feeling and to express it in your work'.

OBJECT:

Finding distraction and relaxation.
Enhancing the moment.

MATERIALS:

Free choice.

INDIVIDUALLY in the Group

EXPLANATORY NOTES:

A relatively brief follow-up discussion is appropriate after completing the work, so that the feeling people had, their experience and what they did with it, stays in the front of their mind. This is more important than the thoughts they may formulate in retrospect.

EVALUATION:

- Were you able to lose yourself in the imagination exercise?
- What sort of feeling did you have during the exercise?
- How did you handle this in making your expressive work? Were you able to hold on to that feeling?
- What materials did you choose, and why?

11.21 ASSIGNMENT 19: Body Image of Emotion

Make a body image of a painful emotion (anger, sombreness, fear, irritability, sadness and so on) in which you show where you experience this emotion in your body, and how.

OBJECT:

Becoming aware of the physical experience of emotions.

MATERIALS:

Free choice.

INDIVIDUALLY in the Group

EXPLANATORY NOTES:

In order to focus attention on the body, you could start with an attention exercise: group members sit on their chairs, relaxed and focus on their body (guided by the therapist). It is important not to be judgemental, but to concentrate on what is observed.

EVALUATION:

- What emotion did you choose to work out, and why?
- How did you develop or represent it?
- Do you recognise the physical experience as a sign of the emotion? Do you make this connection?
- Do you use physical signals as warnings, or how does this work for you?

Reference

Harvey, R., Blum, N., Black, D. W., Burgess, J., & Henley-Cragg, P. (2014). Systems Training for Emotional Predictability and Problem Solving (STEPPS). In C. Sharp & J. Tackett (Eds.), *Handbook of borderline personality disorder in children and adolescents*. New York, NY: Springer.

12

Introduction to Schema-Focused Therapy Module

12.1 Summary of Schema Therapy

Schema-Focused Therapy; A Cognitive Therapy

Cognitive therapy is focused on changing the ways in which people think in order to lessen their mood disorders such as depression, anxiety and anger. Emotions are influenced by cognitive distortions. These distortions are expressed in negative interpretations of, and negative outlooks on, day-to-day events. Cognitive therapy helps clients to change these distortions in their thinking. An important step in this process is looking for evidence of the dysfunctional, unhelpful thoughts. After this, they must be replaced by alternative thoughts that are functional and helpful (Young & Pijnaker, 1999).

What Is a Schema?

If certain thoughts are prominent frequently and over a longer period, we speak of a schema. A schema is an extremely strong conviction held by a person about himself and others that has been learned at a very young age. It often has a self-undermining effect and forms a starting point for a person's thinking, feeling and behaviour. A schema differs

S. Haeyen, *Art Therapy and Emotion Regulation Problems*,
https://doi.org/10.1007/978-3-319-96773-8_12

from other types of thinking in that it is backed by terrific emotional potency of intense lifelong memories that are constantly repeated. Schemas are central to everyone's self-image and world view. A schema has a strong tendency to maintain itself; it can change, or become less powerful, only gradually by actively introducing functional thoughts and new, corrective experiences (Young, Klosko, & Weishaar, 2003).

Functional schemas help people to deal with life in the best possible manner. Dysfunctional schemas form obstacles to flexible and appropriate reactions and pave the way for serious stagnation. They generally do not go away without therapy. Even success in life is not enough to change such schemas. If children, for example, develop the schema that they are incapable, they rarely challenge this conviction, not even as adults.

Even though schemas continue to exist after having been formed, we are often not aware of them. They operate subtly and outside our consciousness. Only when a schema is evoked by certain events do thoughts and feelings become dominated by them. It is precisely at such times that people experience highly negative emotions and dysfunctional thoughts. You could liken it to wearing rose-coloured glasses when a person is in love, which makes everyone and everything seem nice, and wearing dark glasses when you are feeling depressed, which makes everything look sombre and dismal.

Primary Developmental Tasks: How Schemas Develop

Schemas develop in the interaction between a child and his or her environment. If a child is to develop healthy functioning as an adult, he or she has five primary developmental tasks:

- connectedness with and acceptance of others
- autonomy and boundaries
- realistic boundaries
- inner direction and self-expression
- spontaneity and pleasure

When there is optimal interaction between a child and the environment, children develop healthily in all five areas. But when interaction is not optimal, children are more likely to develop early dysfunctional schemas. These schemas are then the organisers of emotional and behavioural functioning. So if there is stagnation in the development of the five developmental tasks, early dysfunctional schemas can arise in the five schema domains on which they are based.

What Are the Schema Domains?

Schemas are found on five domains, corresponding to the primary developmental tasks. In practice, 18 schemas can be distinguished. The book 'Reinventing your life' (Young & Klosko, 1993, 1994) regroups these 18 into 11 schemas or life traps as the authors also call them. Each of the schemas can be traced to the following schema domains.

A. Disconnection and rejection
B. Impaired autonomy and impaired performance
C. Impaired boundaries
D. Overly focused on others
E. Overly vigilant and inhibited.

How Do Schemas Work?

There are three processes by which schemas influence our life and ensure that their presence remains stable:

- <u>Schema confirmation</u> refers to processes by which schemas maintain themselves. The schema will highlight and exaggerate information that confirms it and minimise or refute information that contradicts it.
- <u>Schema avoidance</u> refers to the way in which people avoid activating schemas. This is quite understandable, since schemas can cause extremely negative emotions. There are three ways in which schemas are avoided.
  Cognitive avoidance: Attempts not to think about events that make a person anxious. These attempts may be conscious or unconscious.
  Emotional avoidance: Conscious or unconscious attempts to block painful emotions.

Behavioural avoidance: Avoiding situations that trigger schemas, avoiding mental or emotional pain.

- Schema compensation means exhibiting behaviour that is contrary to what the schema suggests, to avoid triggering the schema. For example, people with a schema of dependence can structure their lives to ensure that they are not dependent on others, even if it might sometimes be better for them if they were. Dependence and counterdependence are very close together, forming opposite sides of the same coin.

Modes

In practice, certain combinations of schemas occur more often. If such a combination of schemas determines behaviour and thinking, we call them modes. There are four types of schema modes:

1. the **healthy adult** mode
2. the **innate child** mode
3. the **protective/maladaptive coping** mode
4. the **maladaptive parent** mode

In each mode, the person has typical thoughts, convictions and behaviour. The same behaviour can occur in different modes and may then have an entirely different meaning. Each mode asks for a specific approach.

In certain situations, modes can be triggered that determine thoughts and behaviour on the basis of earlier experiences. These modes form obstacles to functional reactions in the here and now.

Schema Therapy

Therapy includes attempting to become acquainted with these modes, to recognise them in yourself and to learn to deal with them, in order to arrive at the development of the mode of the healthy adult. Giving schema modes a name and a place (including a historic place) can provide guidance and grip. Therapy is formulated in schema mode terms, focusing on correcting the schemas from childhood (in part by means of limited reparenting) and allowing them to develop, switching off the protective states (because they are dysfunctional) and replacing the internalised parent schemas (which are dysfunctional because they are demanding, punitive or rejecting) by healthier schemas. The fundamental idea of schema-focused therapy is that ultimately, the healthy adult schema will determine the largest part of a person's functioning.

Introductory Module

This introductory module discusses the theory of schemas and offers an opportunity to investigate which schemas are important for each person. This knowledge makes people alert to their own dysfunctional thoughts. The challenge is then to place functional thoughts in a powerful position opposite the dysfunctional thoughts.

Below is a brief introduction to the positions that come forward in borderline disorders and narcissistic disorders. It includes an explanation of the functions of these positions and of the aim of achieving the position of healthy adult. This module is only an initial exploration and provides a framework within which we will look at our own schemas and our own past.

Modes for Borderline Disorders

The following modes are generally present in the diagnosis of borderline disorder:

The detached protector

In this mode, people adopt an aloof attitude to protect themselves against their surroundings. This mode is developed very early as a survival mechanism and its function is self-protection. It is difficult to make contact with others in this mode because these people remain detached and distant. They may experience strong feelings of alienation, in which phenomena such as dissociation and depersonalisation can occur (unconsciously creating so much distance that their own feelings are not readily accessible; this offers protection against painful and sometimes almost unbearable emotions). In this mode or state, people need a calming and safe, secure environment in order to recover so that they can come in contact with their own emotions.

The vulnerable child

In this mode, people feel the earlier pain and grief of being abandoned, in the broad sense of the word, by caregivers. They react as if abandonment is also taking place now, and this forms an obstacle to giving and receiving attention, interest, confirmation and love. People in this mode feel extremely vulnerable, and they primarily need care and attention (not solutions).

The angry child

In this mode, the anger at being abandoned is upfront, and this anger determines a person's entire thinking and behaviour. There is no room for any perspective or reasonableness; the person reacts as if abandonment is taking place here and now. In this mode, a person can fairly easily damage relationships because the emotional response arises from previous experiences and has very little to do with the present. In this anger, which is unreasonable for the situation in the here and now, there is also the wish to punish the other for the suffering inflicted. The environment has much to contend with when a person is in this mode, and may become exhausted or choose to forgo contact if the mode often comes to the fore. In this mode, boundaries are needed in the form of clarity, not punishment. It is important that people learn to channel their own anger and impulsiveness.

The punitive parent

In this mode, people view themselves from the position of a punitive parent and blame themselves for situations. This mode is also developed as a survival mechanism and gives people a sense of control over situations. The child has learned at a very young age to behave well so that dreadful situations no longer occur. The child vents on itself the anger that is in fact meant for the caregivers and the environment. In this mode, people condemn their own behaviour and emotions, forming an obstacle to further development. It is important for a person in this mode, together with a helpful environment, to fight off the punitive parent and send him or her away. This creates room for self-esteem and tolerance of oneself. The requirements that people set for themselves can then be adjusted downward, from an unrealistically high level to a realistic and achievable level.

In therapy, the focus is on learning to recognise and integrate these modes so that scope is created for the mode of the healthy adult. This mode is comparable to the wise mind in Linehan's dialectical behaviour therapy. The healthy adult knows his or her inner child and cares for this child's needs. The healthy adult knows her own painful experiences and feelings, gives them a place and if necessary imposes limits on herself. The healthy adult strengthens his own healthy functioning, reacts as much as possible on the basis of the here and now and maintains good contacts with his surroundings. A person in this mode has self-respect and therefore exhibits good self-care without excessive dependence on others. If the healthy adult is to develop, a period is needed in which corrective experiences take place; this is often done in therapy.

Narcissistic Disorder Modes

In therapy, the narcissistic personality often seems to be the mirror image of the borderline personality. Whereas people with a borderline disorder are needy and particularly sensitive, people with a narcissistic disorder seem to remain insensitive or aloof. The core problem of people with narcissistic disorders seems to consist of the difficulty they have with giving and receiving true, sincere love. The central schemas involve an emotional deficit and a sense of failure. The following modes are generally present in narcissistic disorders.

The lonely child

People in this mode feel inferior, alone and unloved. They feel like a small child, one who is only valued when she does what her parents or caregivers want her to do: Their love or support can only be expected the child shows exceptional performance. This makes it important to continually strive to be the most successful. These people often have the idea that any successes achieved are in fact above their level, and that they can only be thanked to luck and external circumstances. Or they may have the feeling that they can no longer meet expectations, and may well be found out any minute now.

If these people have to rely on themselves, they feel empty and have the feeling that they do not deserve to be loved. As a result, they strive to be unique or special. Being ordinary or average is associated with not being loved, with being ignored. This creates very high-performance standards, and people place themselves under enormous pressure to achieve them. This mode occurs particularly if a special source of status or esteem disappears, such as the loss of a job or a relationship. The mode also occurs when people are confronted with someone who is more successful. Then they have strong feelings of inferiority, failure and loneliness. They will try to escape from this painful mode as soon as possible and move to one of the two following modes. A person in this mode needs acceptance and a sense of belonging.

The overcompensator

People in this mode feel they are better than others. In company, they are demanding, competitive and rude. With this attitude, people overcompensate their feelings of inferiority and failure. They glorify themselves to prove that they are superior, better than all the others. People in this mode are quick to show insensitivity towards others.

Sometimes this includes concealed narcissism. In that case, this mode is expressed in fantasy; people do not openly boast about themselves. For the outside world, they seem to be modest and engaging, but in their fantasies they feel superior to most people. They may fantasise about success and status to be achieved in the future, or about an ideal love affair. In the mode of self-glorification, people often provoke conflict. In such a case, it is important not to become involved but to point this out to them. They must be approached in a clear and non-punitive manner.

The detached protector

People in this mode shut themselves off from their own emotions by doing things that have a soothing, calming effect and distract attention from their emotions. It is a way to avoid the pain of the lonely child. This mode primarily comes to the fore when people are not in company and cannot make an impression on others or be admired by them. In this mode, avoiding emotions can take on many forms, such as seeking stimulating activities (clubbing, sexual contact, sports) or calming activities (using the computer, watching television, fantasising). With these compulsive interests, people distract attention from the pain of the schemas emotional deficit (lack of perceived love and support) and emotional failure (feeling inferior).

The healthy adult

The healthy adult can help the lonely child to feel cherished and protected and let him or her feel love for others. Affection means accepting imperfection, loneliness and the accompanying pain.

The healthy adult makes the demanding self-glorifier aware of his critical, disparaging and patronising behaviour and shows him or her that relationships are not about obtaining approval and admiration; the healthy adult can help the person to develop contacts on an equal footing.

The healthy adult helps the detached protector to give up his avoidance and calming behaviour and helps him or her to be open to love and to experience and express his feelings (self-expression).

12.2 Multidisciplinary Relationships in the Various Aspects of Treatment

Schema Therapy: An Introduction Dysfunctional behaviours are determined by schemas and modes the origins of which are understandable, whereas they themselves are no longer functional. Recognition of one's own behavioural patterns offers scope to make a choice and to learn to deal with situations in a more functional manner. Skills: Recognising and avoiding dysfunctional patterns (pitfalls), practising more functional patterns in thinking, feeling and acting.	
Skills training	Psycho-education: Recognition of dysfunctional schemas and modes. Investigating more functional behavioural patterns, practising them with the aid of a helpful thought
Homework	Working method in behavioural analysis, behavioural experiments
Basic group	Unstructured group in which, for example, members can discuss strategies for dealing differently with recurring situations that are difficult for them
Art therapy	Emotionally ordering and gaining insight into thought patterns and reaction patterns and linking this to the theory on schemas and modes by making expressive works with themes appropriate to adult, parent or child positions, in the self or in contact with others. Although a person's past is considered, the effect in the here and now is the central focus. Looking into and coming into contact with childhood modes Carrying out art therapy assignments in which schemas are activated and behaviour can be practised

Music therapy	Making musical portraits of one another. Attention to how schemas and modes are expressed in playing music together. Magnifying these. Many assignments focused on experimentation
Psychomotor therapy	In the first session, various activities to recognise behavioural patterns and schemas One domain is dealt with in each subsequent session. The idea is to investigate schemas and to experiment with new behaviour
Sociotherapy Starting and ending the daily session/ environment	Completing the schema questionnaire. Discovering themes and explaining schemas when they come up. Systematising the theory, understanding it and learning to take advantage of it. Holding up a mirror when clients are in danger of stepping into a pitfall. Discussing behavioural alternatives and choices they have. Encouraging them to find effective solutions

12.3 ASSIGNMENT 1: Picture of Your Childhood

The therapist instructs:
'Make a picture of your childhood in the way a photograph would have looked at the time. This may be a picture of a real photograph if you have one, but it can also be an image from the past that simply occurs to you. Figure out how old you were then, what you were doing, what your surroundings looked like, and so on.
If you need some guidance, you could make a sort of photograph on a somewhat smaller format (maximum A4) surrounded by a white edge. Use more freedom of expression if you like'.

Here the idea is not to immediately bring up the most difficult experiences, but simply the first picture that comes to mind.

OBJECT:

Becoming aware.
Exploring early schemas and gaining insight into them.

MATERIALS:

Free choice of materials that promote expression, such as drawing and painting materials, paper or clay.

INDIVIDUALLY in the Group

EXPLANATORY NOTES:

This assignment makes a link to the reality of a person's own past. Estimate whether the group members know each other well enough to allow some intimacy.
If you want to increase the degree of structure in this assignment, you can ask for a realistic image or a replica of an existing photograph.

If clients have already learned some theory on schemas, and perhaps completed a questionnaire (YSL), they have been put on track to think about their own schemas. If this is not the case, the therapist should include a bit more theory in the follow-up discussion. This assignment is easily linked to the five primary developmental tasks:

- connectedness with and acceptance of others
- autonomy and boundaries
- realistic boundaries
- inner direction and self-expression
- spontaneity and pleasure

EVALUATION:

- What did you make, and can you tell us something about it?
- What does it mean to you now?
- What is it like to look at this work here right now?
- Which developmental task do you recognise as being related to the childhood picture you made?
- What childhood mode might this be suited to? (Abandoned child, angry child, adapted or free child)

12.4 ASSIGNMENT 2: Working with Clay in the Group

The five schema domains as defined by Jeffrey Young are shown on a flip chart.

A. disconnection and rejection
B. impaired autonomy and impaired performance
C. impaired boundaries
D. overly focused on others
E. overly vigilant and inhibited

The developmental tasks are briefly mentioned, perhaps with some comments or explanation.

A large piece of clay is divided into equal parts among the group members. The idea is that each of them will work this clay individually, without talking, but seated so that they can see each other easily.
The object is that after 10 or 15 minutes, everyone has made the same thing, or at least everyone's work looks as much as possible like the others. It is therefore important to keep looking at each other closely. At the end of the time period, the therapist announces that time is nearly up and that the group must (non-verbally) choose the time when they will all stop.

OBJECT:

Gaining insight into your own schemas.
Experiencing and investigating your own role and attitude in group-focused assignments.

MATERIALS:

1 large piece of chamotte clay, a number of bases to work on, some clay-working tools (optional).

GROUP

EXPLANATORY NOTES:

The assignment can turn out to be quite confrontational because schemas become active and immediately perceptible (see evaluation questions). The internal relationships in the group (which includes any conflicts) will perhaps be openly presented. The group dynamics are clearly perceptible in who takes the initiative, who withdraws, who adapts and so on.

Even though the assignment is to focus on each other, this arouses a wide range of feelings and behaviour: to deviate from this, or to adapt as well as possible to all the others. It also becomes clear how much a person wants to see of himself or his individuality in the work.

Optionally, the exercise can be done a second time, and everyone can choose to practise using different behaviour.

EVALUATION:

For the evaluation, everyone is given pencil and paper. First the group members write down their answers to the questions, and then the answers are exchanged orally. This is so that everyone can first think about their experience during the exercise.

- What was it like to do this, what did you feel?
- What did you see happening in others and in the group; what were important moments?
- Can you link your own experience during this exercise to the domains? Do you recognise your own behaviour in one of the domains?

In the oral part, further questions may also come up such as:

- What took place in the group: Who decided, who followed? How did this take place, and what did you feel like at that time? Did this determine your behaviour?
- Did you focus strongly on the others, or more on yourself?
- Did you sense boundaries, and how did you deal with that?
- What feelings did you have during the exercise? Anger, guilt, shame, concern, anxiety, vulnerability? What schema does this fit in with?

12.5 ASSIGNMENT 3: Big Self and Little Self

The therapist instructs:

1. 'Make a representation of your "big self" in clay; a human figure of how you feel when you feel strong and grown up. You have 20 minutes for this. You may use clay in different colours'.
2. 'Now make a representation of your "little self", a human figure showing how you feel when you feel tiny or unreasonably emotional (for example, whimsical, very anxious or angry). You have 20 minutes for this'.
3. 'Think about what they do with each other, what their relationship is to each other, and bring this relationship to expression by placing them in a certain way relative to each other. You have 5 minutes for this'.

Introduce the assignment step by step.

OBJECT:

Gaining insight into the various positions you occupy as a person.
Gaining insight into what position you generally occupy (what do you show a lot of and what do you show little of?)
Investigating the various needs related to this.

MATERIALS:

Clay, coarse and fine chamotte clay, several different colours.

INDIVIDUALLY in the Group

EXPLANATORY NOTES:

This assignment is well suited to a Gestalt therapeutic framework.

EVALUATION:

- Describe how your big self and your little self look individually. What is important in the way they are given shape?
- What do the two parts of you do with each other? What is their relationship to one another, or how did you place them in relation to one another? Is the distance between them small or large; how would you describe the contact they have?
- Ask about a dialogue between the two of them: 'If one of them were to say something to the other, which of them would say something? What would it say? What would the other reply?' (You may ask them to write this down, so that the words do not disappear.)
- Which of the two sides do you know best; which side do you show more often (group members may give feedback to this)? Which side do you know less well, or show less often?

12.6 ASSIGNMENT 4: Focus on Modes

Brief introduction on the positions that come forward in borderline disorders: The abandoned child, the angry child, the punitive parent, the detached protector. Explanation of the functions of these positions and the aim to arrive at the position of the healthy adult (see the theory in the summary). The clients have this written information and can also read it right now.

'Choose from the written information with the four borderline modes (detached protector, abandoned child, angry child and punitive parent) the mode in which you recognise yourself the most. Work this out in a manner of your own choosing. To offer more structure: First paint a background in two colours, and then work on the basis of the mode you have chosen'.

OBJECT:

Gaining insight into your own emotional and behavioural patterns.
Gaining insight into what mode is most familiar to you, and which one you avoid.

MATERIALS:

Free choice.

INDIVIDUALLY in the Group

EXPLANATORY NOTES:

At the beginning of the task, the written information is handed out, and group members individually link the theory to themselves.

Continuation of this assignment:
From the written information, choose a mode that you are less familiar with but with which you would like to do something (for a subsequent session). Reading the information a second time, group members may discover an underlying mode that was not immediately apparent but which is sometimes primary.

EVALUATION:

- What mode did you choose and how did you represent this?
- What do you recognise of yourself in it, and when does this occur?
- How did this feeling or this behaviour originally arise? How does this affect current situations?
- Was what you represented something you dealt with recently? What was this?
- What is it like to look at it now, with some distance (literally)? What insight does this give you?

12.7 ASSIGNMENT 5: Imagination Exercise, Present and Past

Imagination exercise:
'Sit down where you have enough room so that you can concentrate and are not distracted by others around you. If you like, you may close your eyes. If

you prefer not to close your eyes, just let them rest on a neutral point opposite you. Sit up straight, relaxed, with your legs straight next to each other, feet on the floor under your hips, keep your back straight and don't lean against the chair or table, keep your back straight and imagine that your head is being held up by a thread through the top of your head. Your arms rest quietly on your legs. Focus your attention on your breathing. Is your breathing calm ... is it fast or slow, are your breaths shallow, or deeper, reaching your abdomen? Breathe in and out deeply and try to let your breaths go deeper. Don't be distracted by sounds you may hear around you, just observe and let go of them. Focus your attention on your head and the muscles in your face, try to relax them, or if you like, first tense them and then relax them ... Focus your attention on your neck and feel whether you can relax here too ... Go to your shoulders, feel the tension that may be there, tense up and then relax ... Go to your arms and your hands, tense up and relax ... Focus your attention on your back and your abdomen, feel the muscles and feel how you carry yourself, let this tension relax too ... Go to your legs, your knees, your lower legs and your ankles, tense up and relax ... Now feel how your feet are on the ground, and imagine that you can let any tension you might still feel disappear in the floor ...

Now try to imagine yourself in a **pleasant situation in the present**, one in which you felt very pleasant and safe ... Where are you? ... Are other people with you ... who is there with you? What does this situation look like ... what do you see around you? What do you feel? Is it hot or cold, are there particular smells? Let this situation sink in well ...
And once you have the situation well and clearly in mind, let go of it ...

Now go in your thoughts to an **unpleasant situation in the present** ... When did you feel unsafe, unsure? Are there others with you in this situation? Who is there? Where are you while this is taking place? What is happening, is anything said? What do you feel? What do you feel physically? Are there any other things you notice in this situation?
Once you have this situation clearly in mind, let go of it ...

and imagine yourself in an **unpleasant situation when you were a small child** ... Wait and see if an image comes, don't force it ... Look around you where you are, what does it look like, who is with you - is anyone with you? - and feel how it affects you ... Look at the situation and what is taking place ... and examine what you feel ... and what you think.

Now imagine that you, the **adult who you are now walks into this situation** ... What would you do or say to help yourself as a small child, or to intervene? What could you say or do? And now imagine that you actually do this ... what do you say, or what do you do? What happens, what is the response, or what changes in the situation? ...What do you feel? ...What would you like to do now? Do it, and then what happens? ... Make sure you have said everything you wanted to say. That you have done everything you wanted to do … Is there nothing more you would like to say or do?

Now let go of this situation and go back to the **pleasant situation in the present** … Do you remember where you were? Try to see this situation clearly in your mind again … feel what this situation does to you, what you feel …

….

Now gradually let go of this situation too … bring your attention back to this room; where are you? Do you hear sounds? When you are ready, open your eyes … take your time.

Would you be able to make an expressive work representing part of what you have just imagined? It's up to you which part that will be. Try to keep your attention focused on yourself and not to talk to others'.

OBJECT:

Gaining insight into your own experiences and feelings.
Learning to recognise links between the feelings that play a role in the present and the feelings from the past.
Recognising your own patterns or assumptions.
Working through and changing patterns and assumptions.
Showing yourself in the group in the way you give form to personal experiences and making the group a partner to these experiences and feelings.

MATERIALS:

Drawing and painting materials.

INDIVIDUALLY in the Group

EXPLANATORY NOTES:

If a person is psychotic or has a borderline psychosis, or might decompensate, this exercise is contraindicated. The fear of losing control and being overwhelmed by emotions may be too great, in which case the exercise might increase the person's anxiety. It has been my experience that anxious participants can sometimes benefit when they do not actually take part, but simply observe. This is because in that role, something nevertheless speaks to them and can be developed in their expressive work.

Variations to this assignment:

- Ask group members to represent all parts of the exercise (expanded assignment lasting several sessions).
- Ask them to represent only the part in which they acted as an adult.

The advantage of the form described here, in which group members decide which part of the exercise they will work out, is that a client may make this decision (autonomy) and thus may decide where the boundary is as to how personal it will be. This also makes it clear where a person is in the therapeutic process and what a client intends to achieve in this process.

EVALUATION:

Because this exercise can have great impact and it is important that participants can hold on to their experience, one option is to work with the questionnaire. In that case, everyone can think about the exercise individually before the follow-up discussion. (For the questionnaire, see the annex.)

- How did you experience the exercise; did the images appear on their own; did they halt or falter? What could be the reason?
- What situations and what feelings came forward during the exercise?
- What situation did you portray, and how did you arrive at this choice?
- What was it like to walk into a situation from the past as an adult? What could the adult do, and what significance does this have in the here and now? Is it possible to take care of yourself, to assert yourself, or not, and what does this mean for how you now deal with difficulties?
- How did you portray the situation? What does it look like, and does it evoke the feeling that goes with the situation?
- What feelings or thoughts do you have, looking back? Did you gain more insight into your own feelings, experiences or personal history? What lesson can you take from this, or what did you become aware of?

12.8 Annex Imagination Exercise Past—Present

Questionnaire

Name:

Were you able to relax?

Did the images come of their own accord, and did they slow down or stop somewhere?

What situations came forward and what feelings and thoughts did you have in relation to them?

1.
2.
3.

What situation was the most difficult for you to experience?

1. Pleasant present
2. Unpleasant present
3. Unpleasant past

What did you choose to portray, and why?

1. Pleasant present
2. Unpleasant present
3. Unpleasant past

The reason for this was:

How did you experience it, portraying your own situation, and what strikes you the most in your work and how you represented it (what does the form look like, what feeling comes forward in it)?

What is an important theme for you, and what is an important feeling for you that comes forward here?

What was it like for you to enter the situation from the past as an adult, and what did this do to you?

What feelings or thoughts do you have, looking back?

What has this exercise given you?

12.9 ASSIGNMENT 6: Caring for Your Inner Child

Make an image with the theme of 'your inner child' (25 minutes).
Make something to go with it that the child needs, something that would enable to care well for the child. What would give the child a good feeling? (15 minutes)

OBJECT:

Gaining insight into your own childlike needs (exploring, recognising, acknowledging).
Learning to take care of yourself in the mode of the injured, contented/free, angry, anxious or abandoned child.

MATERIALS:

Free choice, for example clay and other materials.

INDIVIDUALLY in the Group

EXPLANATORY NOTES:

These clients in this group often do not care for themselves properly. The object is to learn to care for yourself and to learn to use this skill mindfully.

EVALUATION:

- How did you give shape to the theme of 'your inner child'?
- What did you make to go with it that would be caring for the child? How does this feel?
- Are you satisfied with it?
- Do you care for yourself in daily situations in this way as well? How do you do this, or why do you not do it?
- Could you decide to do something in this regard, something that is manageable, to put this into practice in the coming week?

12.10 ASSIGNMENT 7: Photograph of Past and Present

Preparation:
Everyone brings two photographs of himself or herself, one photograph from the past and one from the present.

To start off the session, the photos are shown to the group and perhaps briefly explained.

Make a work in which you use the two photos and combine them. In order to work with the photos, they can be photocopied/reproduced on paper or transparent sheets, magnified or reduced. In the work, a relationship or link is shown between the two photographs.

OBJECT:

Thinking about, gaining insight into feelings about your own history.

MATERIALS:

Paper or transparent sheets, photocopies of the photos (magnified or reduced), coloured paper, kite paper.

INDIVIDUALLY in the Group

EXPLANATORY NOTES:

A copier must be available in order to work with the photographs. Many people prefer not to use original photos. When the therapist asks the group to prepare for this assignment by finding useful photographs and bringing them along, the aspect of copying can be mentioned.

EVALUATION:

- What did you do with the pictures you brought with you?
- Describe your work; what did you do, what materials did you choose?
- What is the relationship or link between the two pictures? How did you show this in an expressive work?
- What is it like for you to see this work now, in retrospect?
- What feeling does it give you?

12.11 ASSIGNMENT 8: The Tormentor

The therapist instructs:
'We have all experienced it to some degree: Defeatist thoughts when you are unsure of yourself. You can picture it as a sort of tormentor sitting on your shoulder that comments on the things you do, who says imaginary things that are very negative and self-defeating. Now I want you to give shape to this tormentor. Use your imagination! After that, add text balloons in which you write comments the tormentor could well make to you'.

OBJECT:

Investigating and focusing on self-defeating thoughts and self-image.
Allowing yourself to use your imagination.

MATERIALS:

Drawing and painting materials, paper in several formats.

INDIVIDUALLY in the Group

EXPLANATORY NOTES:

In the follow-up discussion, it may become apparent when this negative self-image, these self-sabotaging thoughts first started. A distinction can be made between the past and the present. What was internalised in the past can now be placed outside of yourself in making your expressive work. This often evokes new thoughts or feelings: Sadness or anger or perhaps just putting things into perspective ('I always think like that, I don't remember when I started doing it, but it is quite strange that I actually started to believe it!').

There is also an 'angel' on your other shoulder, the counterpart to the tormentor, who says kind and encouraging words to you. If desired, this assignment can be expanded to include portraying the angel and adding texts as well.

EVALUATION:

- What does your tormentor look like? And what does it say to you?
- When is the tormentor's presence the greatest?
- Do you recognise the messages from the tormentor as coming from other persons or situations?
- How do the texts or messages gain an influence on you?
- What is it like to look at this work here right now? What do you feel? What thoughts come to mind?

12.12 ASSIGNMENT 9: Meeting in the Woods

Imagination exercise:
'Sit down as comfortably as you can on your chair, with your arms on the arm rests, your feet slightly apart, directly under your knees. You may

close your eyes if you wish. If you would rather not, then focus your eyes on a quiet place in the room – for example, on the floor in front of you. Try to relax the muscles in your face, your neck, your chest, abdomen, back, arms and legs. Then follow your breaths as they go inside, towards your abdomen, and slowly back out again. Follow your breathing again from outside to inside.
Imagine that you are walking out of doors; you look around you and feel the outside air; you are walking along a road and after a bit you find yourself on a sand track. The ground now feels different, and when you look around you see meadows, you hear your own footsteps ... You come to the edge of a forest; you walk on, between the trees, and go deeper into the woods ... It gets cooler and darker; you smell the forest air, the trees, and you hear the leaves rustle. Do you hear a bird? After a bit, the woods are darker, denser with vegetation; your path becomes narrower. After a while you see a light, far away ... you walk in the direction of the light and when you can see it a little better, you see a campfire ... the flames give off a yellow and red glow, they crackle ... you come closer and to your surprise, you see that there is someone by the fire ... that person is someone you know ... he or she has been waiting for you ... you look at the person ... the person says something to you ... he gives you something, you take it ... after a while you say something to the person by the fire by way of saying goodbye and slowly, you retrace your steps. First you walk again through the thick forest where there is very little light ... the undergrowth is thinner and a bit more light and warmth comes through the trees ... you find yourself on the sandy track again and you see the meadows ... you are back on the road, you look around ... and then you are back in this room ... Observe what you now hear and remember what the room looks like. Now slowly open your eyes again'.

Based on the above exercise and the images it evoked, make a visual representation.

OBJECT:

Gaining insight into your own world of experience.
Investigating what schema domain is important or active (see theory).

MATERIALS:

Clay, drawing or painting materials, perhaps other materials that can be combined with them.
Schema domains written on a flip chart.

INDIVIDUALLY in the Group

EXPLANATORY NOTES:

In the imagination exercise, there is a person who is important to the client and has a particular function. This person wants to make something clear, pass on a specific message, by his or her presence, in what the person imparts. This offers the client insight into something that is important to him or her, something he or she may not be fully aware of. This may be related to the schema domains that are important for the client's self-image or world view.

EVALUATION:

- What was it like to undergo the imagination exercise?
- Who did you meet at the campfire and what did this person pass on to you or make clear to you? What took place during this meeting?
- What did you make? How did you arrive at this choice of materials?
- What does your work express? Can you specify this based on the work you made?
- What do others observe in this portrayal? (question to the group members)
- Can you make a link to the schema domains (as shown on the flip chart)? What domain is important to you in this manner of working?

12.13 ASSIGNMENT 10: You and Your Father or Mother

The therapist instructs:
'Make a portrayal of yourself and your father or mother (or another important carer) in which you represent the relationship you had with one of them as it was or still is. Don't make an ideal image, but one that expresses reality as it was in the past or is today. The representation may be figurative or more symbolic'.

OBJECT:

Gaining insight into the significance of the relationship with father/mother for the person's present functioning.
Investigating what schema domain is important or active (see theory).

MATERIALS:

Free choice.

INDIVIDUALLY in the Group

EXPLANATORY NOTES:

The relationship with a father, mother or another important carer (e.g. if the person was adopted or taken into care) is important and formative for the relationships a person has later in life. By investigating these, schema domains that are active become clear, as do possible counter-reactions (schema avoidance, schema compensation).

EVALUATION:

- Did you make a portrayal of the relationship with your father or your mother, and how did you arrive at this choice?
- What was it like to work on this? What did it feel like?
- What did you represent, how did you give it shape?
- What do you think of it when you now look at it with some distance?
- What is the most important theme that comes forward in it?
- Do you recognise this theme as something that you also encounter in other situations or other contacts? How defining is this theme for you? What schema domain can this be linked to?

12.14 ASSIGNMENT 11: The Glasses You Look Through

The therapist instructs:
'The starting point is 'the glasses you look through' as a symbol for how everyone observes and interprets situations coloured in his or her own way. You could compare it to wearing rose-coloured glasses when a person is in love, which makes everyone and everything seem nice, and wearing dark glasses when a person is depressed, which makes everything seem sombre and dismal. Make the glasses you look through and let them show how you observe, and what is characteristic or typical of you in many situations. Make the glasses so that you can actually wear them'.

OBJECT:

Becoming aware of the way you colour your observations.
Gaining insight into the influence of this observation, the colouring or interpretation of your own reality and your own feelings.

MATERIALS:

Wire, chenille yarn, coloured paper, transparent material (transparent sheets, coloured foil), markers, paint, string, beads, feathers, etc.

INDIVIDUALLY in the Group

EXPLANATORY NOTES:

Optionally, clients may make more than one pair of glasses (or one pair with two different sides) to represent duality if they see themselves wearing completely different pairs of glasses.

EVALUATION:

- Tell something about your own glasses; how did you make them?
- What is important about or typical of these glasses?
- Put the glasses on; what strikes you when you wear them?
- What strikes others about these glasses? (question to the group members)
- When do you wear these glasses the most?
- What advantages or disadvantages do the glasses have for you?

If they like, clients may try out wearing each other's glasses, or take pictures of a person wearing the glasses he or she made.

References

Young, J. E., & Klosko, J. S. (1993, 1994). *Reinventing your life*. New York: Plume Books.

Young, J. E., & Pijnaker, H. (1999). *Cognitieve therapie voor persoonlijkheidsstoornissen, een schemagerichte benadering*. Houten: Bohn Stafleu Van Loghum.

Young, J. E., Klosko, J. S., & Weishaar, M. E. (2003). *Schema therapy: A practitioner's guide*. New York: Guilford Publications.

13

Assignments for Special Situations

The underlying assumption is that special situations are important and deserve special attention. A new group member, a conflict or a crisis in the group or saying goodbye are difficult moments, and so they are particularly well suited to practising the skills described in the various modules in the therapy group. Rituals help to shape these moments.

13.1 Multidisciplinary Relationships in the Various Aspects of Treatment

Special situations (new group member, crisis, evaluation, saying goodbye)
The group is supported in dealing with far-reaching events that happen in everyday life, both in the group and outside it, in the personal lives of clients. These situations offer clients opportunities to practise the skills they have learned and to enlist insights in a functional manner.

Skills/goals: learning to deal more adequately with changes and the feelings they evoke, which may be complex

S. Haeyen, *Art Therapy and Emotion Regulation Problems*,
https://doi.org/10.1007/978-3-319-96773-8_13

Skills training	Psycho-education: Continual change is part of life and brings not only confrontation and loss but also opportunities for new development Choices become clear and clients are helped to make more functional choices
Homework	Working method: behavioural analysis, behavioural experiments
Basic group	Unstructured group in which, for example, members can discuss strategies for dealing differently with recurring situations that are difficult for them
Art therapy	When a new client arrives, the group explains art therapy to him or her, and in the first session, this person is given an introductory assignment (not the same assignment as the other group members) If there is a crisis, the group members are encouraged to express themselves about it within accepted frameworks, with the goal of learning to deal with conflict effectively and adequately Evaluations and farewells are marked by giving and receiving feedback, and goodbyes also involve a farewell ritual
Music therapy	Practising playing contrasts and transitions on an instrument. Linking cognition to perception. Composing your own pieces; this is aimed at participating, finding your own basis and making contact with your perception and with others. Seeking your own patterns and playing them
Psychomotor therapy	The group explains psychomotor therapy to a new client In a crisis, clients are invited to make use of a c during the therapy in the psychomotor therapy room When a client leaves, he or she receives a *tableau vivant* (anchor) depicting the group
Sociotherapy starting and ending the daily session/ environment	Assisting and structuring. Providing for transparent rituals in the sociotherapeutic environment that offer grip and structure and in which feelings can be experienced. By repeating rituals, people learn to notice differences in emotions in themselves. Examples: familiarising a new group member with how things work, queuing up to say goodbye, starting and ending the daily session. The sociotherapist lends an ear when there are problems and puts a check on 'ministering' behaviour

13.2 ASSIGNMENT 1. Observation: Introductory Collage

When a client joins an existing group, he or she makes an introductory collage during the first session, while the other group members are given an assignment suited to how far they are in the module.

The new group member chooses pictures and texts from a pile of magazines and makes a collage introducing himself or herself. The pictures and texts can be torn out or cut out, and then glued to a sheet of paper as the person chooses. Coloured paper or drawing or painting materials may also be used.

OBJECT:

Becoming acquainted.
Observing.

MATERIALS:

Magazines, scissors, paper (white or coloured). Optionally, drawing or painting materials.

INDIVIDUALLY in the Group:

EXPLANATORY NOTES:

In the follow-up discussion, contact between the new group member and the rest of the group can be encouraged by stimulating the group to respond to the work.
Points to be observed are: how much the client tells about himself/herself and what sort of thing does the client immediately say a great deal about this, or very little; thoughts or perceptions about the person's collage, dealing with materials, how the work is structured.
As the therapist, you can also make contact with the new client by responding to the work. You can give feedback on what struck you and observe how the group reacts to it.

EVALUATION:

- Would you like to show us your collage?
- Can you explain the work you have made? What did you choose to represent yourself, and how did you make the collage?

13.3 ASSIGNMENT 2. Observation: This Is Me

The texts below are each printed on the top of one A4 sheet of paper and handed out one by one. For each sheet of paper, group members have around 5 min to make their reaction to the text using pencil and crayon. First the paper with the first line of text is passed out; five minutes later, the paper with the second line of text, and so on.

THIS IS ME:
IN THE ABSTRACT, I LOOK LIKE THIS:
SOMETHING THAT HAPPENED IN MY LIFE:
FOR ME, CONTACT WITH OTHERS IS:
MY PROBLEM IS:
THIS IS WHAT I WANT TO DO ABOUT IT:
FOR ME, VISUAL ART IS:

OBJECT:

Increasing spontaneity in actions and reactions.
Charting a number of essential aspects of a person in the therapeutic context (self-image, experiences, social contact, insight into problems, help sought, openness and affinity with art therapy).

MATERIALS:

A4 paper with pre-printed texts, 7 sheets per person times the number of group members.
Assorted drawing materials.

INDIVIDUALLY in the Group:

EXPLANATORY NOTES:

This assignment is suitable when an entirely new group starts out or when a large number of the group members are new. The assignment is done with the entire group at the same time, but each person works individually.

This is a fast-paced assignment; clients scarcely have time to think about the questions. It calls upon their direct and spontaneous reactions.

EVALUATION:

- What was it like for you to do this exercise and to work under time pressure?
- What did you do with each sheet of paper, and would you like to say something about it?

13.4 ASSIGNMENT 3. Observation: Human Figure in a Circle

The therapist instructs:
'Make a drawing of a human figure in a circle. How you do that is up to you'.

OBJECT:

Becoming aware of and gaining insight into a personal theme or into how the client assigns meaning.
Observing the manner in which clients make their expressive works, and how much they communicate with each other (consciously or subconsciously) within the remit of the assignment.

MATERIALS:

Pencil, coloured pencils, crayons or charcoal.
A compass or a circle to trace, if wished.
Paper (A4 or A3 format).

INDIVIDUALLY:

EXPLANATORY NOTES:

The human figure may symbolise the person.
The circle can have many meanings in the work, both pleasant and unpleasant—as locking in, as the personal space, as infinite, as a peephole or as an inner world in contrast to the outer world (outside the circle).
A deliberately created picture shows, for example, what a person wants to communicate. A picture that simply developed can unintentionally or unconsciously show specific personal content.

EVALUATION:

- What did you do with the prerequisite of 'a human figure in a circle'?
- Describe the human figure you made; what else can you say about it?
- What is the function of the circle in your picture?
- What is the most important theme in the picture, and is it something you are familiar with?
- Did you want to include a particular meaning in your picture, or did it find its way there unintentionally?
- What do you think of this picture?

13.5 ASSIGNMENT 4. Observation: Boat on the Water

The therapist instructs:
'Paint a watercraft on the water. This can be just about anything: a boat, a freight ship, a sailing boat, a rubber boat, a nutshell, and so on. Make it any way you want. The water on which the boat is floating can also be just about anything. It can be a lake, a sea, a bathtub, an ocean—it's up to you. You may combine painting and drawing materials'.

OBJECT:

Gaining insight into the client's issues and how he or she feels about life right now.

MATERIALS:

Paint, soft pastels and oil pastels.
Paper, 50 × 65 cm.

INDIVIDUALLY in the Group:

EXPLANATORY NOTES:

The elements in the picture are regarded as symbols by means of which the client communicates something about himself or herself, whether deliberately or not. The boat symbolises the client. The water may show how that person feels about life in general.

The assignment can be given at the start of treatment because it may make quite a lot clear about a client. For a group that has been together for some time, this assignment can be given as a group task, in which the boat symbolises the group.

The degree of insight obtained depends on the links made in the follow-up discussion by clients and/or the therapist.

EVALUATION:

- What kind of boat did you make? How is the boat painted? How big is the boat?
- Is there land in sight? What is the weather like? How is the water? What direction is the boat going, and is this with a tailwind or against a headwind?
- How important are the surroundings?
- What does the boat say about you?
- Do you recognise the circumstances the boat is in?

13.6 ASSIGNMENT 5. Crisis: Picture of the Group

If there is an argument or if there are problems between members of the therapy group, have the group members each make a picture of the group showing how they see or perceive the group right now.

OBJECT:

Learning to analyse a problem in the group.
Participating in and investigating conflict.
Expressing your own opinion.

MATERIALS:

Free choice.

INDIVIDUALLY in the Group:

EXPLANATORY NOTES:

In such a crisis, it is important to link the behaviour of group members to their individual treatment goals. By offering this as an individual assignment, everyone's standpoint and everyone's perception comes forward. In a group discussion of a conflict, there are often several group members who contribute actively. In this assignment, each group member is involved and sets to work. Group members cannot hide, or in any case, have much less opportunity to do so.

In the follow-up discussion, a link can be made to dealing with conflict situations in general, or in earlier situations. It is important to ensure that there is a focus on feedback to the present situation, and what people do with that right now.

In a conflict in the group, the therapist has a psycho-educational role; you show that you make problems open to discussion, and how that can be done in a respectful and effective manner. You may have to be more directive than otherwise.

EVALUATION:

- How did you portray the group, and what does this show about how you feel in this regard? Make sure that each group member has a chance to have their say!
- Is your present manner of dealing with this conflict the same as or different to what you have done in the past? (What is old behaviour, and what is new behaviour?)
- What does this conflict say about you as a group?
- What do you do too much of, and where do you do too little?
- What do you resolve to do in future?

13.7 ASSIGNMENT 6. Crisis: The Wailing Wall

Hang a large sheet of paper, perhaps brown packing paper, on the wall. The group is told that this paper is a wall on which they may write down anything that bothers them: free and uncensored, the lot. Imagine it to be the fence people write on at night, when no one is looking.
The group will first have to do something with the paper so that it looks like a real wall. After that, they can vent their frustrations on the wall. As the therapist, you encourage everyone to have a turn and ensure that people really let off steam.

OBJECT:

Expressing and venting dissatisfaction.
Making dissatisfaction open to discussion.

MATERIALS:

A large sheet of paper, perhaps brown packing paper. It must be really big. Depending on group size.

GROUP:

EXPLANATORY NOTES:

This assignment is appropriate if there is much unexpressed or undifferentiated dissatisfaction in the group, but it is mainly projected outside the group, and from a therapeutic point of view, you want bring it out in the open.

EVALUATION:

- Who wrote what on the wailing wall? Can you explain a bit?
- Do you recognise things that others wrote on the wall? Do you agree with everything?
- What was it like to do this assignment?
- What do you as a group do with this dissatisfaction?
- What do you resolve to do?

13.8 ASSIGNMENT 7. Evaluation: Reflection—End of Module

Think about what was the most important for you in the past weeks in relation to emotion regulation/crisis skills/interpersonal skills (depending on which module precedes this).
What have you learned? What have you discovered about how you can handle emotions or situations differently, or better? Portray this in your own way.

OBJECT:

Exploring, recognising and acknowledging what you have learned.
Holding on to, defining/specifying and confirming positive learning experiences.

MATERIALS:

Free choice.

INDIVIDUALLY in the Group:

EXPLANATORY NOTES:

Reflection, thinking things over and having an overview are generally quite difficult for this group of clients. They tend to live in the moment, to be awash with emotions or to focus on the here and now. This assignment asks clients to look back and to see what was the most important thing they learned. It may be no more than an insight, a piece of knowledge that has not really been put into practice yet. It is important that they realise this as well. You can help clients to explore, to recognise and to acknowledge what they have learned by together discussing the past weeks and the effects of the issues that came up in their treatment. The picture they make here lets them hold on to these aspects. It makes the work they have made something almost real; it anchors and confirms what they learned as the basis.

EVALUATION:

- What was the most important learning experience for you in this module?
- How did you portray it?
- How do you think you can ensure that you can hold on to this discovery, to what you have learned? (Take a picture of this work, take your work home and put it somewhere where you will see it?)

13.9 ASSIGNMENT 8. Evaluation: The Central Thread

The therapist instructs:
'From the works you made during your treatment period, choose the three most important ones (for any reason whatsoever) and put them in front of you. Based on these works, how do they show the central thread in your process, or how do they fit into this process?

On this basis, make a new work, in which you may use features or material from the three previous works. This new work is focused on the central thread in your process'.

OBJECT:

- Evaluating the client's own process.
- Self-insight, insight into the therapeutic process.
- Anchoring the therapeutic process by making clients more conscious of it.

MATERIALS:

Free choice.

INDIVIDUALLY in the Group:

EXPLANATORY NOTES:

On the basis of a client's own works, this assignment helps them to get a grip on the expressive therapy process and to hold on to it. Starting from this basis, they can determine new goals.

EVALUATION:

- What three previous works did you choose and why did you choose these particular ones?
- What was the most important aspect of expressive therapy in the past weeks?
- How have you portrayed it now?
- How does it feel to reflect back on this? Is it confrontational, or confirming?
- What are your goals for the time to come?

13.10 ASSIGNMENT 9. Evaluation: What Do You Take with You—What Do You Leave Behind?

Everyone takes a black marker and divides a sheet of paper into two equal halves.
On one half, they draw a large circle. This represents a waste bin viewed from the top.
On the other half, they draw a large square with a handle. This represents a bag.

The therapist instructs:
'Think about the most recent period, and decide for yourself what you want to leave behind and what you will take with you. Using drawing and painting materials, make pictures of what you want to leave in the bin. In the bag, make pictures of what you want to take with you'.

OBJECT:

Evaluating.
Making choices about holding on to and letting go of experiences and behaviours.
Promoting exchange in evaluations and making choices.

MATERIALS:

White paper 50 × 65 cm, black marker, drawing and painting materials.

INDIVIDUALLY in the Group:

EXPLANATORY NOTES:

This assignment encourages clients to express themselves clearly about a previous period, in which both positive evaluation and critical evaluation are given a place. Clients are also asked to look ahead, to where they will have to choose what they want to keep.

EVALUATION:

- Explain what sort of work you made; what do you want to leave behind; and what do you want to keep? What does it look like?
- Do the other group members recognise this? Had they expected you to make this choice?

13.11 ASSIGNMENT 10. Goodbyes: Farewell Ritual

When a person leaves the group, the following farewell ritual is carried out in the last session.
Group members make something for the person leaving. It portrays what they will remember about the person leaving and what they want to give that person to take with. This may be positive, but it can be critical as well.

The group can also decide to make a shared work in which each group member makes a separate part.

The person leaving makes something for the group members based on the same theme: What will stay with you about the others, what do you want to say to them?

OBJECT:

Taking leave purposefully by focusing on it in the form of a farewell ritual.
Recognising, describing and dealing with emotions in relation to leave-taking.
Learning to accept the feeling of being left behind or abandoned, and expressing it in a careful and mature manner.

MATERIALS:

Free choice.

GROUP/IN PAIRS/INDIVIDUALLY

EXPLANATORY NOTES:

During their treatment, group members experience this ritual a number of times. This means that they will know what will take place during their own leave-taking, it is a goal to work towards.
Some clients dread the ritual because they are the focal point, and they perceive thinking and talking about taking leave as something extremely difficult. They prefer to simply gloss over it. But generally speaking, in the end, the experience is very positive, and in retrospect, prized, perhaps even cherished. It gives people a good feeling to take part in the farewell ritual, and it has a positive after-effect.

The therapist has a participating role in this ritual and also makes something for the client that gives concluding feedback. In the follow-up discussion, the therapist has a coaching role and sets an example for group members. The phased follow-up discussion is important here because it leads up to focusing and reflecting on the act of taking leave.

EVALUATION:

In the evaluation, the person leaving is the first person to receive anything; this is a deliberate choice. All group members are invited to talk about what they have made and their experience of the farewell ritual. It is important that they do this directly, that they tell the person leaving and personally hand over what they have made (not simply push it across the table). When the person leaving has received everything, the therapist asks how he or she experienced receiving works, so that the experience, the feeling is acknowledged and talked about.

The final step is that the person leaving gives the group members what he or she has made and tells them the message it has for them.

Annex 1

The Strength of the Expressive Medium

The strength of the expressive medium is defined here as the therapeutic effect the art medium can have. Whether it actually has this effect depends on several factors, including the therapeutic relationship and the client's motivation. The strength of the art medium lies in a number of aspects related to working expressively—the activity itself—and the resulting work.

The strength of the expressive medium lies in:

- **The creative nature of expressive work**

  The client makes something. This experience shows clients that they can have an influence on materials and perhaps, looking a bit further, they realise that they can have an influence on their surroundings. In brief, clients can become aware of their own influence and can feel for themselves that they can make something that that is theirs, and theirs alone.

S. Haeyen, *Art Therapy and Emotion Regulation Problems*,
https://doi.org/10.1007/978-3-319-96773-8

- **Simply working creatively**
  Working creatively is largely guided by unconscious motives. The process itself can have a positive effect. It assumes that clients are active.
- **Patterns and mechanisms in working expressively**
  Clients have different manners in which they make an expressive work. Some clients will first sit and think for quite a while, working something out completely in their mind, and then simply produce it. Other clients may quickly make something, and then keep changing it until they are satisfied.
  There are also very different ways in which clients deal with an impasse, when they can get no further in the expressive process. How a person works gives you essential information about how that person deals with things, such as problems, resistance or dealing with others.
- **The individuality of the visual language**
  We identify ourselves with what we see. For example, we fly when we see a seagull flying, or in other words, we empathise with the things or shapes we see.

What makes the visual language powerful? Several aspects can be distinguished; they can be seen directly in the work.

- **Colours**: Colours can have a warm or a cool effect; often, too, an emotional expression, such as soft or bright. A colour can take on a symbolic meaning: red, for example, means anger. What feeling or atmosphere does the work exude?
- **Form**: Forms can be very different: closed, erratic, geometric, round, enveloping.
- **Lines**: Every line has certain characteristics, such as straight, curved, short, long, dynamic, slack, shaky or angled. What do the shapes and lines say?
- **Unarticulated form elements**: These are the unplanned details that wind up in the work, such as scribbles that look almost accidental.

- **Composition and the relationship between the visual elements**: Is the composition static or dynamic, orderly or disorderly? A disorderly composition may point to an inability to structure, to a sense of being overwhelmed by emotions, or capriciousness. How is the work constructed? Is it stacked, for example? Is one element the most important, or are all of them equally important? Does one element push another off the paper, so to speak?
- **Handling the materials**: What kind of the texture does the work have on the outside? For example, is it finished roughly or smoothly? This says something about how it was made and it gives the work a certain manifestation. Were mixed or unmixed colours used?
- **Function of the expressive work**: Is it an example of self-expression; is it meant to be useful, or is it basically decorative?
- **Content/meaning/theme**: Working with a large format, bigger movements can be made than on a small format, which asks for a more restrained, controlled manner of working. A large art work stands out more. Choosing a large format can sometimes serve to gain attention.
- **Level of detail**: If a person shapes a work elaborately and with extreme care, then he or she is probably very much focused on technique or appearance. This may have to do with a need for control, of wanting to be in charge, or wanting to make an impression on others.

  Together, these areas of visual language constitute the **expression**. The strength of the visual language is what it says about the person who made it, or what the work said to him or her. This may be more than what the maker wanted to show: it may say more about the maker than the person intended to tell.

– **The expressive medium as a learning tool, to practise on**

The expressive medium offers many opportunities for practice, experimentation with conduct or new behaviour. An example: Try to let yourself be led by coincidence, whereas you would otherwise anxiously avoid anything like this. You can learn something from it.

- **A material, a tool or a theme can hold an appeal for the client**
  A working material, tool or theme can exude a powerful appeal. Clay, for example, has a particular sort of attraction. How does the client respond to this? Clay invites you to squeeze, smear, knead. It is in the material itself. One client will lose himself completely in working the clay by squeezing and kneading, while another will try to make perfectly straight-lined geometric shapes and minimise physical contact with the material. Do clients let the material define them, or are they eager to do that themselves? Here the strength is also found in the fact that as the therapist, you can utilise this: you provide one material and not the other, which allows you to observe how a client deals with what the material says, while the client can acquire new experiences with different approaches.
- **The product of the expressive activity**
  The product provides a **visible and tangible result** of what took place in the activity. It is easy to look back; it is all identifiable.
  The product asks the client to **adopt an attitude**. What does a person do with it? Is it cherished, cultivated, or is it made to look ridiculous? Does one client allow herself to bond with it, does another simply break the contact?

Two perspectives for expressive therapy treatment:

1. **The manner of working and the product say something about the maker.**
   The expressive work communicates a particular meaning and sometimes shows more than the maker was aware of wanting to show (it acts as a mirror or self-image). Through the expressive work, clients communicate about personal themes and they gain insight by reflecting on their own work and its meaning. Clients can use aspects they have become aware of as they continue the expressive process. From this perspective, emphasis is on aiming for **awareness, insight into and processing** their problems (leading to a change in the person). Some aspects of the strength of the expressive medium that come forward here: the individuality of the visual language, patterns and mechanisms in expressive work, what sort of appeal the medium has, and the final product.

Questions in this regard are: What strikes you about the expressive work, what recurs over and over, what is always absent? How does the client perceive the expressive work and what meaning does it have for him or her? How does it relate to their personal problems or needs? From this perspective, it is primarily about emotional significance and meaning.

You can use what the work says, the character of certain elements it contains, to raise awareness in the client. In the follow-up discussion, you can try to discover what the work means for the person who made it, and you can place the therapist's vision of the work alongside it. Differences between them can be a valuable source of information or exchange.

2. **The expressive medium as a learning resource, something to practise with to arrive at new behaviour**.

   Clients can practise and experiment in dealing with certain things and in expressing themselves. From this perspective, emphasis lies on **internalising the expressive work process and skills** (leading to a change in behaviour). Aspects such as creating an artwork as a means to practise, the product, patterns and mechanisms in working expressively and appeals made by the product come forward here. In these aspects, you see how clients work, how they conduct themselves in working with the expressive medium. Behaviour and product are central. In this manner of working, we look to see if similarities, analogies can be found between a client's manner of dealing with and working with the medium and his or her problems. The therapy can simply focus on an expressive problem without trying to gain insight.

Annex 2

The Pictures File

The pictures file contains a wide range of photographs and pictures from magazines, newspapers, books and so on. The file is a rewarding source of inspiration and has plenty to offer when preparing assignments. This file can also help a client actively come up with ideas.

Possible categories of pictures:
Women
Men
Relationships
Homes
Pictures of nature/landscapes
Animals
Inspiration
...

S. Haeyen, *Art Therapy and Emotion Regulation Problems*,
https://doi.org/10.1007/978-3-319-96773-8

Some assignments that make use of the pictures file:

- Giving and receiving feedback (Crisis skills 3)
- Making choices (Emotion regulation 21)

Some other possible thematic ideas for assignments:

- Your problem is … (for a group member)
- My relationship
- Ideal house
- The group as animals

Annex 3

Three product descriptions that relate to varying degrees to clients with personality issues, depending on the seriousness of the problems and the further issues: 'Focus on self', focusing on trauma and autonomy, an eating disorder and a module focused on learning to express feelings.

FOCUS ON SELF

Trauma treatment and recovery of autonomy in expressive group therapy

Care programme: Anxiety disorders

Working method: Provides focal insight

S. Haeyen, *Art Therapy and Emotion Regulation Problems*, https://doi.org/10.1007/978-3-319-96773-8

Rationale	Clients with traumatic experiences have suffered extreme damage to their sense of autonomy. They are often unable to integrate the events in their mind and have not yet been able to talk about them. Working expressively provides a way to set this process in motion. This applies in particular to persons who have a difficult time findings words for their experience or for persons who can put it into words, but who are unable to come in contact with their own feelings
Indications	Traumatised clients, with DSM classifications of post-traumatic stress disorder or an acute stress disorder, both type 1 and type 2, with one or more of the following symptoms: • Inability to integrate traumatic, stressful experiences in their daily life • Feeling dependent on others • Inability to deal with conflicts and/or conflicting feelings • Suffering from their own survival strategies/techniques that are aimed at not feeling pain and grief
Contra-indications	• If, as a result of giving expression to the trauma, the client feels completely overwhelmed and the symptoms worsen • If there is a chance of psychotic decompensation • If clients are unable to watch or listen to other group members
Objectives	General: • Increasing or restoring autonomy Specific: Clients learn: • to act and to remain active • to give direction to their own acts • to integrate traumatic or stressful experiences • to act on the basis of daily reality rather than on the basis of the traumatic or stressful experience • to know their own individuality and to appreciate it in their daily existence

(Continued)

Interventions	Seeking the individuality in the person's expressive process or what is characteristic of his or her work and following it throughout the process, expanding or strengthening it. In the works made, the personal experience or the trauma will generally be the starting point The process and the pace are largely determined by the client; clients choose their own route. The therapist calls on the client's autonomy as much as possible and when necessary, offers guidance and structure. The first time, making a lifeline is frequently taken as a starting point, after which it can be worked on as part of a process. The therapist offers assignments or materials, makes suggestions or offers support, but the client's own choice is decisive. The therapist creates conditions, asks questions to clarify matters and gives feedback or psycho-educational explanations Follow-up discussions and evaluations over a longer period are important so as to give words to the experiences and to the works, to keep objectives clearly in focus and to view the process from a greater distance, establishing a link to the trauma. The works and the experiences in therapy are the guidelines for discussion. Assignments are both supportive, with much explanation, pacification and psycho-education, and ego-strengthening, with supportive and structuring elements, and/or aimed at cognitive changes
Conditions	Further training in trauma treatment Half-open group with limited intake
Subtypes	Gender-specific groups for men or women only Individual therapy
Treatment duration and frequency	Weekly sessions of 75 minutes, maximum duration is individually determined (target period nine months)
Attainment targets	The client has increased autonomy to the extent that: • he/she can actively guide his/her own conduct • the traumatic experience has been integrated in a way that it no longer dominates daily functioning (conduct, thinking and feeling) • the client recognises, experiences and appreciates himself/herself more, which is expressed in aspects such as behaviour and acknowledging and giving expression to his/her own opinions and wishes

Art therapy eating disorders group

Care programme: eating disorders
Working method: Provides focal insight

Rationale	Clients with an eating disorder or characteristics of an eating disorder are often trapped in a pattern of acting and thinking. A negative self-image lies at the basis. This is expressed in finding it difficult to be visible as an individual, impaired contact with emotions, experiences and cognitions and impaired social contacts. The art therapy eating disorders group focuses on these aspects by making expressive work and discussing it and through their contact with each other
Indications	Clients with an eating disorder, anorexia nervosa or bulimia nervosa, or with characteristics that show a strong tendency towards avoidance behaviour, rationalisation and/or perfectionism with little self-structuring ability. They can profit from the presence of group members. Age categories: adolescents (to age 23) and young adults (20–35)
Contraindications	If the eating disorder is so predominant that the person can no longer profit from the group and the presence of group members
Objectives	Learning to let go of rigid behavioural patterns Ending their isolation Restoring contact with their own emotions, experiences and cognitions (both in relation to the eating disorder and to the underlying problems) Visualising their own problems, accepting them and learning to deal with them

(Continued)

Interventions	Working with expressive materials where the expressive work serves as a transitional object, thus improving their contact with their own needs, making them visible. Connectedness and giving up isolation are central to showing the work and talking about it. The expressive product offers an opportunity to take some distance and acts as a mirror, providing a concrete reality test In art therapy, both the route (the process) and the expressive work (the product) are central. The use of various materials suggests to clients that they should improve contact with their own needs, perceptions, experiences and cognitions. This is the process-oriented step The next step is to actively give shape to the experiences and visualise them in an expressive product. Because the resulting product is tangible, clients are confronted with their own functioning and they are able to take some distance and to adjust, accept and deal with cognitions, emotions and perceptions The working method in this group is ego-strengthening, with supportive and structuring elements, and/or aimed at cognitive changes such as focusing on insight, working on resistance and interpreting transference
Conditions	
Subtypes	This group is offered as part of an outpatient eating disorder programme and further comprises a verbal therapy group and psychomotor therapy
Treatment duration and frequency	Weekly session of 75 minutes, maximum duration nine months. Every six weeks there is an entry and an exit moment; it is a half-open group
Attainment targets	Clients have gained insight into their own behavioural patterns, and insight into their own emotions, perceptions and cognitions. Clients have developed a more positive self-image and are better able to enter into contacts. The eating disorder has disappeared into the background or has decreased and can be dealt with better

Art therapy group 'LEARNING TO EXPRESS YOURSELF'

Care programme: mood disorders/personality disorders
Working method: insight-plus

Rationale	In this therapy group, clients who rationalise a lot and for whom this has become part of their disorder have an opportunity to open themselves to expressive work and to the group members so as to have more emotional contact with what it is that causes them to get stuck. Expressive work offers a completely different way to make contact than does talking This product also concentrates on clients who have difficulty in regulating their feelings, meaning they are often quite intense. On the basis of specific assignments, working expressively offers clients a way to compare themselves to others and helps regulate them
Indications	Adult clients (aged 25–55) with high-level cluster B or C personality disorders who have one or more of the following symptoms: • Mood disorders such as mood swings or persistent sombreness • Tendency to avoidance • Vague physical complaints • The feeling of being stranded, stuck • Burnout complaints • Tendency either to rationalise or to drown in emotions
Contraindications	Chance of psychotic decompensation The risk of being completely overwhelmed by what takes place in expressive therapy and being unable to remedy this or deal with it. Insufficiently willing to learn by doing and experiencing Inability to profit from the presence of group members
Objectives	Learning to express themselves Learning to set boundaries Learning to share experiences with others Coming in contact with their own feelings Coming in contact with others Gaining insight into their own emotional and behavioural patterns

Interventions	*Role of therapist*: The therapist adopts a supportive, structuring attitude and offers insights. Resistance and transference are interpreted and processed. The working method is ego-strengthening and focused on cognitive changes *Activity*: The expressive therapy offers room for the issue a client wants to look into, while structuring the assignments, interventions and follow-up discussion. An equilibrium between expression and structure is the aim Contrasts in perceptions, thoughts, elements of the work, making the work and symbols are worked out and both aspects are visualised so as to create coherence and integration The follow-up discussion is used to give words to experiences, to keep the objectives clear and to view the process from a distance *Materials*: A wide range of materials and assignments with great expressive possibilities can be used which can be completed within one or two sessions. The use of all kinds of scribble/spatter techniques and assignments that invite clients to work spontaneously and without a plan fits in this programme
Conditions	An experienced therapist is needed to oversee and steer the processes
Subtypes	
Treatment duration and frequency	Weekly session of 1 1/2 hours in an open group composed of both men and women. The duration is individually determined based on the treatment goals and is a minimum of three months and maximum of two years
Attainment targets	• Clients allow themselves to express what occupies their mind, are not afraid to show themselves • Clients experience their own feelings and investigate their own behaviour without fleeing from it • Clients enter into contact with others, allow themselves to share experiences and maintain this contact • Clients have gained insight into themselves • Clients also know how to impose limits on themselves

Index

S. Haeyen, *Art Therapy and Emotion Regulation Problems*,
https://doi.org/10.1007/978-3-319-96773-8

H

I

L

The manufacturer's authorised representative in the EU is Springer Nature Customer Service Centre GmbH, Europaplatz 3, 69115 Heidelberg, Germany. If you have any concerns regarding our products, please contact ProductSafety@springernature.com

Printed and bound by CPI Group (UK) Ltd, Croydon, CR0 4YY
25/09/2026
02222852-0002